MINDFULNESS

THE MAGIC OF LIVING IN THE PRESENT

The Simple Art of Practicing Gratefulness To Achieve Happiness and Peace

MADELINE CHAPMAN

Table of Contents

Introduction

Humans, at the core, are energetic beings. Throughout our lives, it is very easy for our energies to become out of balance due to traumatic events, grief and loss, and daily stressors which are often a result of unhealthy societal and cultural expectations. If you look closely at yourself and other people and feel like something seems to be missing, the information in this book is for you.

This book will address three parts of the whole which are crucial to healing the entire being on an energetic level: Mindfulness, Chakras, and Energy Healing. Each section will be followed by Guided Meditations and Journaling opportunities so you can adequately process what you are learning and keep track of how it impacts your experience. Additionally, the book contains a toolkit of 50 mini-meditations to give you a place to start and keep you on track in your journey. The information within these pages will demonstrate the flaws in the general population's approach to health; true healing is not possible without understanding all parts of the whole. This book will describe what healing looks like on a molecular level and revolutionize the way you consider health and healing. You will be given all the tools you need to check in with yourself, monitor and nourish your energies, return to the present moment, heal from the pains of your past, and ultimately, return to your highest self.

PART I

Section 1: Mindfulness

Finding Your Way Back to the Present Moment

Chapter 1: Back to the Basics

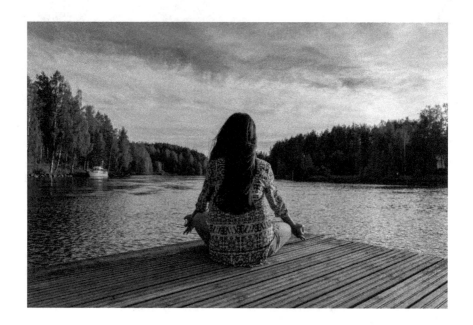

When most people think of mindfulness, they envision monks or yogis, sitting cross legged for hours with closed eyes and poised fingers overlooking the Himalayas. Although mindfulness is present in the lives of monks and yogis, what most people don't know is how easy it is to incorporate mindfulness into our everyday lives. As a matter of fact, a mindful state is the most natural and restful state for human beings—a state in which we were all living and moving in as children. If you think back to your childhood, you will likely remember that your concept of time and perception of reality was much different. Most children are very in touch with their emotions, letting them come and go naturally. If a child falls down in one moment and skins their knee, the child will likely begin to cry. However, if a few moments later they are being offered ice cream, their tears will dry, and they will continue on with their day. Mindfulness is the reason children are so in tune with the details of life that adults seem to miss. It is also the reason they are more likely to screech with joy, run around excitedly in enjoyable environments, wake up easily in the morning, and take the time they need to calm down from anger or sadness until the next happy moment arises. Children spend very little time thinking about things beyond the present moment. Even if they have something to look forward to, they are still likely to become invested in the moment at hand, whether that is playing, enjoying time with their parents, or eating a meal. So, what happens as people grow older that brings us away from this natural state of mindfulness?

There are a number of factors that pull people out of the present moment. From the time a child begins elementary school, they are presented with a schedule for the day, which remains relatively the same. Children are expected to remain within the structures presented to them, and the idea of forward-thinking and preparing for the next hour's activity becomes introduced. As they grow, children will likely have more expectations placed upon them, whether those expectations are academic, extracurricular, or within the home. Of course, it is necessary for children to learn how to be responsible and dedicate the time they need to the important things in life. However, as they become further exposed to the constant rush and future-oriented thinking of their parents and teachers, they come to see time as something that no longer belongs to them to fully inhabit.

Furthermore, as people approach teenage and young adulthood, they will begin to face challenges that most children are either shielded from or otherwise unaware of. People become flooded with the pressure to perform well and always be doing more today than yesterday. Although the expectations of cultures and societies vary, we can be sure that people are overwhelmed with the pressure to meet those expectations in order to be considered successful and valid. Once one bar is crossed, another one is waiting, and there is no time to slack. Additionally, the older people become, the more likely they are to be subject to long-lasting pain in their lives. This can come in the form of relationships ending, failing to accomplish something, being mistreated by other people, losing and grieving loved ones, or coming to terms with painful childhood events that did not make sense at the time. Teenagers become increasingly subject to mental health issues as they advance into adulthood, having to face all of the hard realities of the world and still come out on top. People may also be subject to trauma as a result of illness, accident, or abuse. All of these factors are enough to work against people and pull them out of the present moment, either because it is too painful to be there, or because they are simply too distracted.

Human beings experience over 60,000 thoughts per day, but the vast majority are dedicated either to planning for the future or worrying about the past. Becoming overly concerned about the future or steeping in the pains or regrets of the past can increase levels of stress in the body, which makes people more anxious and prone to physical health problems.

The mind naturally wanders, and it is impossible to keep thoughts from coming. Mindfulness is not a tool to eradicate such thoughts, as is the common misconception. Rather, it is a tool through which to acknowledge the thoughts the mind creates, bring attention to them, and allow them to move through. This ultimately brings people into what is happening here and now and gives them more control over their minds and how they orient themselves in their environments.

Because mindfulness is a skill that all human beings are equipped with at our core, it is something that can be re-learned. Just as we exercise our bodies to strengthen our muscles, so we must work to strengthen our brain through mindfulness. The way this strengthening happens is through being aware of thoughts as they arise, then breathing back into the present moment. The more practice is given to returning to the present moment, the stronger the mind will become in remaining in the present more often. Just as the body physically strengthens and becomes healthier over time with exercise, mindfulness exercises can physically change the structure of the brain to make it healthier. Mindfulness activates the positive components of the hippocampus, which is the part of the brain responsible for good things like creativity, joy, and the ability to process emotions. This, in turn, decreases stress levels, depressive tendencies, addictive behaviors, and the fight or flight instinct by shrinking the part of the brain responsible for negative things (the amygdala). Overall, increased mindfulness is the key to a longer, healthier, more creative, and more joyful life.

Chapter 2: Unlocking Your True Purpose Through Mindfulness

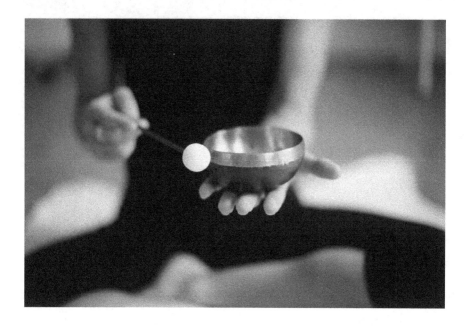

Re-centering Yourself

Everyone has days where everything seems to be spinning out of control, and there seems to be no way to manage the chaos. The days where you wake up late, run late to work, spill coffee on your shirt, get cut off on the road, get yelled at by your boss, spend the entire day at work in a confused frenzy, only to come home and bicker with your partner. Since the beginning of time, the human mind has been conditioned to release stress hormones and illicit the fight or flight instinct for the purpose of protection and survival. In the past, this primal instinct was very useful for escaping threats. As times have changed, the threats have become less severe, but the brain's response has remained largely the same. Now, these fight or flight reactions are likely to be triggered by everyday scenarios, such as those previously detailed. The hormone-induced responses that occur when we're stressed out are quick to send us spiraling into emotionally dramatic, and far less peaceful dimensions.

The good news is, mindfulness can be used as a tool for re-centering and gaining control over your anxiety and emotional reactions when you start to feel yourself spiral. Although there is no way to avoid stress and drama in daily life, mindfulness can serve as a shield of calm presence to protect your well-being. If you are preparing to enter a situation that you anticipate could be stressful, like a high-stakes day at work, a scary doctor's appointment, or a difficult conversation with a loved one, it can be incredibly helpful to bring yourself down to a more calm and balanced state in preparation for the stress you are about to deal with. You may find yourself with a racing heart, sweating palms, an unclear head, and the feeling of "butterflies in your stomach." Another area where it is common to feel these physical effects of anxiety is when encountering dramatic situations. Drama can arise tense moments with other people, as well as within the theoretical situations people create for themselves when worrying about what they cannot control (for example, the perception other people have of them, or events that may or may not occur in the future). Giving attention to what is happening in your mind and body and allowing yourself to breathe into the moment can be a total lifesaver in moments of drama or stress. Two to three minutes of deep breathing in your car before going to work, or taking a few deep breaths before reacting in a tense moment, can make a drastic difference in your sense of balance and your ability to deal with stress without launching into fight or flight.

Giving Your Emotions Space

The goal of mindfulness is not to eliminate emotions, but rather, to gain control over the impact they have on how we orient ourselves in the world. It is vital to honor our emotions and give them space to exist and teach us, without letting them seize control. Mindfulness is an excellent tool for giving our emotions space in this way. When an emotion arises, mindfulness gives us a chance to observe that emotion without judgment. In this calm space, we can ask our emotions, "What are you trying to teach me?" We can more clearly discern why we are experiencing a certain emotion, and become in touch with the deeper needs that may have caused that emotion to arise. Just as a child may cry when they need to be nourished our held, we may find ourselves growing angry or agitated when we need support, touch, or self-care. Similarly, we may find ourselves feeling stressed or anxious in scenarios that are subconsciously triggering moments from the past. In these cases, our stress and anxiety are begging us to become in touch with our past self, reminding ourselves that we are safe, and the traumatic moments from the past are over. Once our emotions have been given a non-judgmental space to exist, they can smoothly and peacefully move through the body and be released. This frees us to move from moment to moment like children do, without being constrained by unresolved emotions. Additionally, giving this space to our emotions in mindfulness helps to temper our reactions, which can prevent us from acting out in extreme ways and potentially doing or saying something we regret.

Making Clear Decisions

With the human mind constantly being muddled with thoughts, it can be hard to see things clearly. Sometimes our minds are cluttered by the expectations flying at us from every different direction, or perhaps by our fears of what will happen if things don't go to plan. When it comes to making decisions, we are often faced with numerous options, and it can be difficult to navigate through the chaos in our minds to come to a well thought out resolution. In a distracted, anxious, or removed state, our minds are like a pond on a rainy day—rippling to a point where there is no more clarity. Mindfulness is the calming of the waters, which brings us to a place where we can more clearly think of all possible outcomes of a decision and check in with what we truly need before moving into the next moment.

Keeping Yourself Safe

Although fight or flight instincts originally developed as a way to keep humans safe, in many modern-day scenarios, they do quite the opposite. Let's go back to the example from the beginning of the chapter about the chain of events in a typical chaotic day. If you wake up late in the morning and rush to make your coffee, not paying attention to what you are doing, you run the risk of haphazardly screwing the lid on your to-go cup, then sloshing boiling hot coffee over the edge of the cup and onto yourself as you bolt out the door. Although such a scenario could simply result in a stained shirt, the inattentiveness could have a more drastic effect, such as burning yourself or someone else. Driving to work in a state of panic over running late causes you to be more likely to break the rules of the road—driving too fast, making dangerous decisions when changing lanes, taking turns too fast, running yellow lights just before they turn red, etc. Additionally, the panicked state can lead to anger with yourself or others on the road, which can further impair judgment and put you at greater risk of an accident. Attempting to have a conversation with your boss if you are in fight or flight mode could result in being overly emotional and saying or doing something extreme which could place you at odds within your workplace, potentially even costing your position. Going throughout your day in a frenzy causes you to be less aware of what is going on around you, which can lead to further threats to safety like leaving a burner on, forgetting to eat or drink enough water, or neglecting those in your care (such as pets or children) as a result of your own inner distractions. Finally, as stress from the day carries into the home at the end of the day, it can pose a major threat to relationships. The more stressed out and less clear thinking you are, the more likely you are to say or do something threatening to your partner, to put yourself in an aggressive and volatile situation, and to make brash decisions that have the potential to haunt your future.

Just as we must give ourselves space to learn, grow, and process our experiences, we must give that space to those around us as well. When a partner or friend is acting in a way we don't enjoy, mindfulness can allow us to take a step back and look at the situation from a position of empathy. We can allow ourselves to hold space for whatever that person may be going through individually and express our support while also maintaining boundaries and staying in control of what we can. Everyone is deserving of space to be listened to, understood, and supported for who they are. However, it is incredibly difficult to give that space to anyone if it has not been cleared within oneself.

When we operate out of a mindless state, there is hardly any space to meet our own needs and process our own experience, much less to provide that to other people. This can lead us to be closed off to the ones we love, push them away, or act out in anger, selfishness, or aggression. If we have not given space to what is going on within us, we cannot offer full empathy to others. Only 20% of the population is recorded to practice true empathy, which can be linked to the rarity of true mindfulness among adults. Mindfulness allows us to be more present to our own needs in order to hold adequate space for the needs of others as well.

Attention and mutual respect are core elements of every functional relationship. Practicing mindfulness can improve relationships with all the people in our lives by preparing us for every engagement and calming our minds enough to be fully present in the moments we share with others. Mindfulness clears the space for us to listen intentionally to other people and pay more attention to what kind of people they are and what kind of support they need. It allows us to love other people better by increasing our awareness of how they feel most loved. By being present in the moment at hand, as opposed to trapped in the past or future, you are more likely to remember to pick up the phone and give your grandmother a call, to be fully engaged when interacting with your child, or to remember the kind of kombucha your significant other likes best from the store. Not only does mindfulness allow for more meaningful conversations and joyful memories, but it also increases the functionality of our relationships overall so that both ourselves and those we love are feeling fully respected, listened to, and encouraged.

Fostering True Joy

We often hear the term "childlike joy" to describe moments of pure bliss, enthusiasm, and full satisfaction. As people grow into adults, such moments tend to be few and far between, with many remembering the most joyful moments to have been those that occurred in childhood. The expectations of daily life become too much, and most people find themselves trapped in a cycle of constant anticipation. People spend so much time thinking about where they would rather be (on vacation, in bed, enjoying the weekend) that the days melt into each other without us realizing all the moments of our lives we are missing. The biggest societal misconception is that true happiness lies in what we do not yet have. We are flooded with lies such as "Once I can buy this new TV, then I'll be happy," or, "Once I have a partner, then I'll be happy," or, "I'll be happy once I can say I've been to five different countries." Mindfulness abolishes these lies by proving to us that the capacity for true joy lies not in the future but in the here and now. Wherever you are right now, whatever you have, and whichever stage of life you're in, mindfulness reminds you that *this* is your chance to experience beauty and satisfaction like never before. Take time to look at the flowers you did not notice growing in front of your neighbor's house, the complexity of coffee's flavor as it slides down your throat, the way your loved one's eyes crinkle when they smile, the laughter of a child, every intricate flavor of dinner, or the unique people wandering up and down the streets you drive every day to work. It is here that joy resides; all you have to do is be present enough to recognize it.

Chapter 3: Moving Mindfully in Daily Life

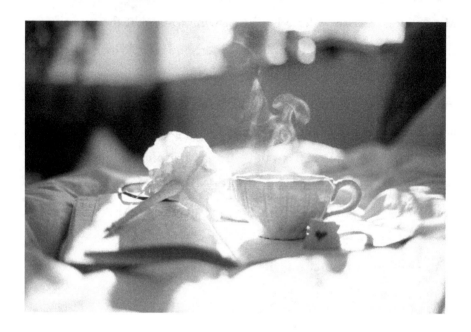

Coming to the Present Moment: Daily Guided Mindfulness Meditation With Journaling (Week 1)

Cultivating Mindfulness

This meditation should be done in a space where you feel fully comfortable, safe, and relaxed. Perhaps it is in a corner of your bedroom, in a garden, by your favorite lake, or even in your car. Make sure you can fully relax and avoid distractions. Some people meditate best with instrumental music or nature sounds in the background, while others prefer silence. Feel free to try multiple methods and see which is most soothing to you (this can vary depending on the day). You may do this meditation sitting in a chair, on a mat, or lying flat on your back with your palms up to the sky. You will need to give yourself 5-20 minutes of time to practice, depending on your skill level and current state. If you like, you can set a timer.

Start by coming into the moment with a few deep breaths. Settle into your body and take note of any sensations you feel. If you feel pain, tingling, warmth, or tightness in any part of your body, focus your breath into that space. Imagine any tension unfurling into openness. Notice as your thoughts arise. Take notice of them, then allow them to pass as you come back to the breath. If it is helpful, you can try a breathing pattern in order to culminate focus. To do the 4-4-4 breathing pattern, breathe in for 4 counts, hold for 4 counts, and breathe out for 4 counts. To do the 5-5-7 breathing pattern, breath in for 5 counts, hold for 5 counts, release for 7 counts. Sometimes it helps to imagine breathing in the things you wish to see more of in your daily life (creativity, love, patience, openness) and exhale the negative things (fear, negativity, sadness, stress). Allow yourself to spend a few moments in a more active state of breathing in, releasing, and paying attention to your body.

With practice, you may enter a state where your thoughts slow and you become fully grounded in the present moment. In this state, you are no longer bombarded with thoughts, nor distracted by elements of your environment. It becomes easier to return to the breath. All restlessness and tension in the body seem to melt away, and the mind reaches a flowing, liquified state. There may be days when you cannot enter into this state, and you remain restless throughout the course of the meditation. If this happens, allow it to be that way, observing every thought that arises, then letting it go.

After the time is up, begin to arrive in the moment by moving your body slightly—wiggling your fingers and toes, tensing and releasing your muscles, etc. Next, you're your eyes. Notice how bright and clear the world looks to mindful eyes. Notice the calm, transcendent feeling in your body, and continue to move with it as you go about your day.

Mindfulness Meditation Journal Prompt (Week 1):

What did you feel in your body before beginning? What do you feel now?

Which thoughts continued to arise in your consciousness? Could these thoughts have been trying to teach you something or speak to a deeper need you may have?

How does the world look after opening your eyes? What do you notice?

Come back after going about your day for several hours. Did you bring mindfulness with you into the world? If so, how?

Coming to the Present Moment: Daily Guided Mindfulness Meditation With Journaling (Week 2)

Taking Mindfulness Into the World

This meditation will be done with your eyes open in moments if your daily life. This is not a specific meditation you have to set aside time for, but rather a state you come into. Notice where your attention goes in a given moment. If your attention is drawn to a particular sight, like the nearest tree or a view from the top of a mountain, allow yourself to see it fully. Repeatedly tell yourself, "see, see, see." Breathe as you allow your eyes to truly become totally focused and take in the image fully, allowing it to become a part of your awareness.

If your attention is drawn to an auditory experience, such as the sound of cars on a city street, a rushing body of water, or an internal monologue, give full attention to that thing. Soak in that auditory experience, breathing slowly and telling yourself, "hear, hear, hear."

You may also be drawn to a particular physical or emotional experience within the body. This experience may be positive, like a pleasant bodily sensation or a feeling of joy. It may also be negative, like physical pain, or feelings of anger or feel. Either way, allow yourself to become fully present with what is there, breathing into the experience and seeing what it has to teach you. Breathe into that bodily experience, telling yourself, "feel, feel, feel."

Throughout the day, you'll find that your attention is pulled in various directions. Mindfulness is the choice to tune in to whichever place you're going in a given moment and give full attention to that experience for whatever it is.

Mindfulness Meditation Journal Prompt (Week 2):

How difficult was it to bring mindfulness into your daily life in this way? Where did you face the most challenges?

Did your attention tend towards certain experiences (visual, auditory, bodily) more than others?

Describe a specific moment where you brought mindfulness to your experience and felt truly present. What did you observe?

Coming to the Present Moment: Daily Guided Mindfulness Meditation With Journaling (Week 3)

Mindfulness at Work (or School)

The first part of this meditation should happen in a place outside of work, where you feel safe, calm, and separated from the issues you may face in the workplace. Start by identifying your biggest struggles at work. The journal portion will give you a space to write them down. Do you struggle with productivity? Boredom? Stress? Conflict resolution? Work relationships? Once you have identified your most significant area(s) of struggle, close your eyes and visualize what that unpleasant experience looks like. Perhaps it looks like you, rushing around mindlessly like a bee in a hive, stressed out and too overbooked to step away and breathe because there are more calls to make, more e-mails to send, more things to do. Or, perhaps it is the co-worker, professor, or boss that makes your stomach drop whenever you think about having to interact with them. Perhaps you feel unfulfilled at work and find yourself constantly checking the clock, thinking about the moment you get to leave. Maybe you have so many things to do and no idea where to start, so you waste a lot of time on mindless tasks. Whatever your struggles at work are, use your time and space away from work to safely visualize the situation. Breathe into the mental circumstance.

As you breathe, begin to envision what this experience would look like if it went the way you want it to. Perhaps it looks like the mental clarity that allows you to know exactly what needs to get done and how to make the best possible use of your time. It could be a greater sense of calm and courage when talking with your difficult boss or co-worker and having your message be well-received on their end. It may also be a deeper sense of satisfaction and enjoyment in the work you're doing, providing you the ability to step back and feel a sense of joy with where you're at, without constantly thinking about the next thing. Reframe the moment in your mind until you've created a mental space that feels good. Let yourself sit there, breathing, soaking it in for several minutes.

Once you go into the workplace (or school), you can bring this meditation into your life by going back to the peaceful mental image you've created over and over again. When you begin to feel stressed, bored, anxious, or unproductive, return to the space where you do not feel those things. Bring that energy into your daily work life, and watch how it revolutionizes your experience.

Mindfulness Meditation Journal Prompt (Week 3):

What do you identify as your biggest challenge(s) at work or school?

How does it look when you reframe your struggles to create a positive mental image?

What do you observe about bringing this positive mental image into difficult situations in the workplace or at school?

One-Minute Mindfulness

- Find a space where you can be alone, like on your bathroom break or in your car right before going into work, school, or home at the end of the day.
- Set a timer for one minute
- Close your eyes and focus exclusively on your breathing
- Take notice of the stresses, thoughts, and anxieties that arise, then let them go
- When you open your eyes, notice how you feel de-stressed, clear-minded, and prepared to go about your upcoming tasks and interactions with others

5-Minute Body Scan

- Set a timer for 5 minutes (if needed)
- Close your eyes and take several deep, cleansing breaths. You may use the 4-4-4 or 5-5-7 breathing patterns to deepen the breath
- Begin to bring attention to your body
- Take notice of any sensations that arise-- warmth, tingling, tension, etc.

- Bring your attention to the soles of the feet. Tighten your muscles by curling your toes, then release. What sensations do you feel?

- Continue moving up the body to your calves, hips, abdomen, chest, hands, arms, face, and neck. Observe any sensations that arise, and breathe into those sensations.

- Tighten and release the muscles in each of these areas, allowing any pent-up energy or resistance to be released

- Feel your body become grounded, relaxing completely into the floor, bed, or chair as you come into the present moment in your body and all tension melts away

Mindful Bath/Shower (10-minute meditation)

- As you begin your bath or shower, take a moment to breathe. Remove yourself from the stresses of the day and allow yourself to re-center

- Bring attention to each part of your body as you wash it

- Take notice of any sensations you feel as you move from the soles of your feet to the ends of your hair

- Breathe in the pleasant scent of the soaps and the warmth of the water. Allow yourself to feel clean, warm, and safe.

- As you wash each part of your body, thank it for what it does for you. Then, thank yourself for taking care of your body.

Mindful Morning Routine (15-30 minutes)

- Before getting out of bed, begin to stretch gently, letting thoughts come and go as your mind and body wake up. Do not rush yourself.

- Once you are ready to get out of bed, bring your attention to the space around you and the day ahead. Feel yourself become fully present in that space and prepared to move mindfully through your day

- Pay attention to every move you make, from putting on clothes, to washing your face, to setting the water on the stove to boil.

- Cultivate your awareness for the day ahead by moving slowly and calmly, one task at a time, becoming fully awake to the world

Mindful Housekeeping

- Allow yourself to become focused on the task at hand and only that task. Let every other thing you have to do or think about fade into the background.

- Bring your attention to the breath and the specific way your body moves as you complete a particular task or chore

- Give space to any thoughts or emotions that arise in your consciousness, allowing yourself to process them in a mindful state

Mindful Sit-and-Drink (10-minute meditation)

- Find a calm, quiet space where you can sit and observe the world around you (preferably outside or near a window looking outside)

- Pour a glass of your favorite tea, coffee, or cocktail to enjoy

- Eliminate all distractions. Draw your attention to the intricate flavors of the drink, and the pleasure of pulling something you enjoy into your body

- Take notice of the things happening around you. Find the things in the environment that bring you the most peace, and allow their presence with you to help you calm your mind. Become completely indulged in the moment.

Mindful Scheduling (10-minute meditation)

- Sit down with a pen and paper and center yourself with five deep breaths.

- Think about the days to come. Consider your priorities, remembering that every task is significant and an opportunity for increased mindfulness

- Ask yourself, "Am I giving myself adequate time to bring mindfulness and intentionality into each of these activities?"

- Take notice of any activities you feel you won't be able to be fully present for. Consider taking a thing or two off the list and saving them for a better time.

- Take notice of any feelings of stress, nervousness, or rush you feel in regards to your schedule. Breathe into those feelings.
- As you continue to write your schedule, allow yourself to feel empowered, in control, and prepared to be mindful of everything you are about to do

Mindful Driving

- Leave the house with plenty of time to be relaxed and focused. After entering the car, take a few moments to breathe and center yourself
- Once you start to drive, begin to take note of the things passing by. What do you see today that you did not see yesterday?
- Breathe in your visual surroundings, using them to center and remind yourself: "I am here. I am in this community. This is my life, and I am awake to it."

Mindful Walking (10-20-minute meditation)

- Choose an area where you can relax and bring attention to your surroundings. This can be in a park, in the city, on the beach, in your neighborhood, etc.
- Set out on your walk with no distractions
- Take notice of the things your eyes fall upon. If something specific catches your attention, allow yourself to pause and breathe it in.

- Pay attention to the sounds that surround you, giving yourself space to truly hear them
- Pay attention to the feeling of your feet on the pavement, the swing of your arms at your sides, and the rhythm of your breath
- Let your heart expand in curiosity and openness to whatever is ready to meet you in this space
- Allow yourself to become totally saturated with your surroundings, remembering that everything you see, hear, and feel is a part of you

Mindful Cooking and Eating

- As you enter the kitchen to prepare food, take a moment to center yourself in the moment with a few deep breaths
- Give every moment of the cooking process your full attention, from washing, to cutting, to cooking. Become fully immersed in the process (you can do this even with simple meals, like mindfully spreading peanut butter on bread)
- Breathe loving-kindness into the cooking process, remembering that the food you make will provide nourishment to yourself and others
- Once the food is ready, clear the eating space of distractions. Avoid multi-tasking
- Chew every bite of food 20-30 times, letting yourself be engulfed in the flavor and practicing gratitude for the nourishment
- Walk away from your meal feeling truly nourished and renewed

Mindful Waiting

- The next time you're trying to distract yourself at the doctor's office, the mechanic, or waiting for a friend or colleague to arrive, remind yourself that waiting is one of the most sacred times to engage in mindfulness

- Breathe into the moment, becoming aware of what surrounds you

- Bring awareness to your body. How are you feeling? Take note of any sensations

- Become aware of the thoughts that come once you stop numbing yourself with distractions. What things are running through your mind?

- Pay attention to the deeper thoughts you may have previously been ignoring. Ask yourself what you can learn about yourself and your life, or if there are any actions you need to take.

Mindful Creativity (at least 5 minutes)

- Set aside anywhere from five minutes to several hours of undivided time

- Engage in a creative project like art, writing, dancing, etc.

- Bring full presence to the creative project and try to eliminate all expectations. Allow the moment to carry you.

- Pay attention to how your mind and body react as the moment carries you. How do you feel?
- Examine what you create as a result of this free-flowing creativity

Mindful Play

- Dedicate time each week to doing something truly fun— something that makes you feel like a kid again (climbing a tree, swimming in the lake, drawing with chalk, baking cookies, having a game night, etc.)
- Eliminate all distractions and allow this to be a moment to step away from your everyday life and responsibilities
- Allow yourself to become lost in the childlike joy of play. Laugh loudly, let your body dance, be curious.
- Let the feeling of childlike joy saturate your body and carry this joy with you as you move back into your daily life.

Mindful Movement (10-30 minutes)

- Choose one of your favorite forms of movement (swimming, walking, dancing, going to the gym, etc.) and dedicate at least ten minutes to it

- As you begin to move, establish a deeper sense of body awareness. Pay attention to the feelings in your body as you begin to warm up and exercise

- Pay attention to the way your heart beats, your lungs heave, your face begins to sweat, and your body tingles with the sense of being alive

- Thank your body for all it does for you.

Mindful Listening/Quality Time

- Apply this meditation to any quality time you spend with another person, whether that is grabbing coffee or going for a walk with a loved one, interacting with co-workers, are conversing with the grocery store cashier

- Before interacting with others, bring attention to your levels of empathy. Set the intention to hold space for other people and the moments you share with them

- Eliminate distractions (like technology) and allow yourself to put everything else going on in your life on pause in order to be fully present

- One of the best ways to show love for people and to cultivate personal mindfulness is through mindful listening. Focus all of your attention on the other person and what they are saying. When you ask how their day is going, be present to hear the answer.

- Do not think of what your next move will be, what you will say, or where you will go. Simply be there, showing loving-kindness, holding space, and taking it all in.

Mini Meditation Toolbox: 10 Quick and Easy Meditations to Ease Stress, Depression, Addiction, Anxiety, Pain, Distraction, and Loss Using Mindfulness

Journaling the Consciousness (10-minute meditation)

- Sit down with a journal and a pen and set your timer for 10 minutes
- As thoughts, worries, or emotions arise, immediately write them down. Do not worry about structure, grammar, or content, just write.
- When the time is up, look over what you wrote
- Ask yourself which themes seem to reoccur. Where are you feeling stress in your life? What is occupying most of your mental space?
- Close your eyes and take a few moments to breathe and meditate on the thing(s) that need your attention the most
- Open your eyes. Notice how you feel lighter and in touch with your experience

Distraction Cleanse: Clearing the Space in your Mind

- *Find a quiet place and begin to breathe*
- Ask yourself: "What is distracting me from being present right now?"

- Give space to that distraction, whether it is an invasive thought, personal emotion, or someone else's emotion
- Say to yourself: "I am letting my distractions move through me as I ground myself in the present moment. Nothing is more important than right now."
- Breathe until you feel the distraction melt away into presence and mental clarity.

Re-Writing the Moment: A Short Meditation to Ease Emotional Pain of the Past

- Sit down with a journal and a pen and set your timer for 1 minute
- Take this 1 minute to write down any moment(s) of the past which have caused you a lot of pain
- After the minute is up, choose one of the painful moments, close your eyes, and begin to imagine the moment in a safe way. Be sure to keep breathing.
- When you open your eyes, take your pen and paper and re-imagine the painful moment. What do you wish had happened? How do you wish you could think about the moment now?
- After re-imagining the painful moment, remind yourself that this is a new moment. Everyone has painful memories, but you do not have to stay in spaces of the past, which are painful for you.
- Close your eyes, take a few more breaths, and say to yourself, "I release the pain of that moment of the past. This is a new moment, and I will move with it."

Re-claiming your Inner Power: A Short Meditation to Face Addiction

- Breathe into the moment, allowing yourself to think about the implications your addiction has on your life

- Without judgment, question your addiction. Ask yourself, "What has been left empty in me that I am trying to fill with this?" Listen for any emotions or past experiences of trauma, grief, or abandonment that arise. Allow them to be there.

- Say to yourself, "Now that I understand the root of my addiction, I can begin to be set free."

- With closed eyes, begin to breathe. With each breath, imagine your addiction's hold on you weakening and weakening until eventually, you have been released.

- Move forward into your life with the idea that your addiction's hold on you is loosening, day by day.

Letter to the Lost: A Short Meditation to Address Grief and Loss

- Sit down with a journal and a pen and take five deep breaths to bring you into the moment

- Allow someone you have lost to come to mind. This can be a relationship that has ended, someone who has died, etc.

- Close your eyes and breathe into the space this person has left empty within you. Allow yourself to experience any emotions that arise.

- When you open your eyes, take a few minutes to write what you wish you could have said to that person

- After you have finished your letter, close your eyes again. Tell your grief that it is okay for it to be there. With every breath, imagine yourself moving forward in your life, released from every regret you may have with someone you've lost

In with The Positive, Out with the Negative: A Short Breathing Technique

- Find a comfortable space and prepare to use the 5-5-7 breathing technique

- Breathe in for five counts and think of something positive you want to bring into this moment (kindness, peace, wisdom, etc.)

- Hold for five counts, allowing this positive thing to fill your body

- Exhale for seven counts, thinking of something negative you want to release from your body in this moment (stress, tension, selfishness, etc.)

- Begin again with a second emotion. Do this as many times as you like until you feel well-equipped with positive emotions and have released all negative ones

Space to Breathe: A Short Meditation to Gain Control over your Anxiety

- When you begin to feel anxious, step away, take a breath, and ground yourself in the moment by finding one thing you can see, one thing you can hear, and one thing you can feel. Focus deeply on each thing.

- Allow your anxiety space to exist. Remember, anxiety is the reaction your emotional brain has when it senses a threat. You can bring yourself back from catastrophe mode by using the rational brain to repeatedly remind yourself: "I am safe. I am in control. I am capable of being calm."

- Keep breathing and saying these rational-brained affirmations until you begin to feel your anxiety melt away

- Move into the next moment feeling calm, anxiety-free, and empowered

Emotion Coding: A Short Meditation to Bring you in Touch with your Emotions

- Find a quiet, comfortable place where you can easily connect with yourself

- Close your eyes and breathe deeply (you may use a breathing pattern if desired)

- Begin to travel inwards. Say to yourself, "I am ready to accept the emotions that are here."

- Wait patiently, focusing on the breath, and observing every emotion that rises to the surface.

- When an emotion arises, ask yourself a series of questions:

  1. "Is this emotion mine or someone else's?"
  2. "Does this emotion serve me or hold me back?"

3. "What is this emotion trying to teach me?"

4. "Should I release this emotion or put it into action?"

- When it comes to answering each question, listen to your intuition. The answers to each question are already within you. Do not question your natural answers.

- If you are being told to release an old or negative emotion, or an emotion that belongs to someone else, breathe and imagine it melting away with every exhale

- If you are being told to foster a positive emotion or a strong emotion that can create positive change in the world, sit with that, breathing, and being open to how that emotion can be useful.

The "I Love..." Gratitude Meditation (2-minute meditation)

- Find a private space, preferably one in front of a mirror

- Start a timer for 2 minutes

- For two minutes, speak out loud sentences of gratitude beginning with the words "I love…" ("I love my partner," "I love coffee," "I love my cat," "I love sunflowers," I love my mom," "I love to dance," "I love that I am healthy,").

- Say as many things as you can, one after the other. Do not think too much, simply let the things you love flow from your lips

- When the timer goes off, look in the mirror and say "And I love you," to yourself

- Feel the magic of gratitude transforming your life, your self-confidence, and your ability to be mindful

The Mindful Manifestation: A Short Meditation to Manifest what you Want in Life

- Sit down with a journal and pen
- Begin to cultivate mindfulness by bringing attention to your breath and any sensations in your body
- Ask yourself the question: "What do I want most in life?"
- As the answers start to come, open your eyes and begin to write your desires with the words "I manifest…" in front of them ("I manifest empathy." "I manifest peace of mind." "I manifest protection." "I manifest safety." "I manifest love." "I manifest awareness." "I manifest wisdom." "I manifest pure joy.")
- With each manifestation, close your eyes, and say it to yourself at least three times. Feel this manifestation become a part of your reality.

PART II

Section 2: The Chakras

Understanding How Energy Functions in the Body

Chapter 4: Essentials of the Seven Chakras

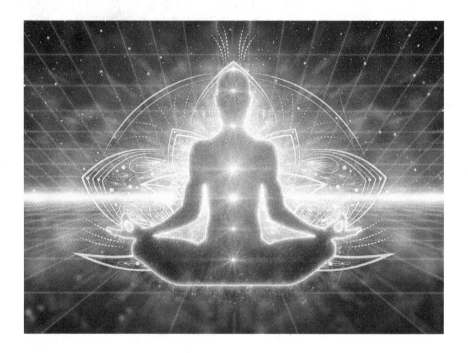

The seven energy centers of the body, labeled by Eastern spiritual traditions as the "chakras" are located in various places along the spine, ending in the brain. They are strongly tied with emotions, instincts, the experience of consciousness, and the experience of love. Each chakra represents a specific area of the human existence and levels of physical, spiritual, emotional, and psychological balance. In order to apply any of the chakra balancing techniques, it is crucial to understand the concept that human beings are composed of pure energy—the same energy that courses through all other things on earth. Although there are different methods for balancing each chakra individually, there are several commonalities in the process of chakra balancing. When a chakra is considered "out of balance," that means that energy has become trapped somehow, which can cause emotional, psychological, physical, or spiritual blockages that can manifest as a variety of health problems. The level of balance of each chakra is believed to correspond to human actions, feelings, health, and general orientation in the world. In this chapter, we will be breaking down each of the seven chakras and what part they play in the whole of human existence.

Crown Chakra

Color: Auric white or violet

Location: Top of the head

Basic Description: Sometimes called by the Sanskrit name "Sahasrara" or "thousand petals," the crown chakra is known as the chakra, which connects to transcendence, consciousness, and connection with the infinite. The location at the top of the head seems to elongate this chakra to the higher source, and all that lies beyond our daily distractions and ideologies. The Crown chakra works closely with the pituitary and pineal glands, as well as the hypothalamus to regulate the endocrine system. This chakra impacts the brain and nervous system and, therefore, can have very direct impacts on a person's state of mental health.

In Balance: When the Crown chakra is well balanced, people are likely to experience feelings of bliss, unity with all that exists, and transcendence in which all limitations are no more. They will feel fully present and aware of the sacred nature of all of life. They become aware of all that lies beyond the constraints of space and time and draw closer in every moment to pure spiritual ecstasy, divinity, and universal consciousness.

Out of Balance: Imbalances of the Crown chakra can manifest psychologically as schizophrenia and delusion, depression, insomnia, and Alzheimer's. On a physical level, it can cause nerve pain, chronic headaches, and disorders of the thyroid and pineal glands. Emotionally, it can manifest as disconnection from the body, the earth, and the spirit, over obsession with spiritual matters, a cynical attitude, isolating oneself from others, and general close mindedness. It can cause a general inability to set or follow through on goals and produce a feeling of lack of direction in life.

Third Eye Chakra
Color: Indigo

Location: Brows; between the eyes on the forehead

Basic Description: Sometimes called by the Sanskrit "Ajna," meaning "perceiving," this chakra is the center of human intuition, as well as human imagination. This energy center is driven by foresight and openness to life.

In Balance: When the Third Eye chakra is in balance, the rest of the chakras are likely to be well-balanced as well. This is because the Third

Eye chakra is seen as a culmination of all other elements in their most pure and balanced form. According to yogic metaphysics, a balanced Third Eye chakra allows for people to transcend the "I" concept and begin to see themselves as deeply connected to the rest of the world, as opposed to separate from it.

Out of Balance: Imbalances in the Third Eye chakra are less likely to manifest psychologically than imbalances of the crown chakra are. However, an imbalanced Third Eye chakra can lead to extreme physical side effects. The relationship to the pituitary gland and general neurological function can lead to decreased metabolism, weakened ability to fight infection, and insomnia. Additionally, a person suffering from an imbalanced Third Eye chakra may experience high blood pressure, seizures, chronic sinusitis, poor vision, migraines, or sciatica. At the most extreme level of imbalance and physical unhealthiness, stroke or blindness can occur. Emotionally, an imbalanced Third Eye chakra may manifest as increased self-doubt and loss of direction in life. People will lose touch with their intuition and, therefore, completely lose sight of their understanding of life and their visions for themselves. They may become paralyzed in moments from the past or terror at what the future may hold.

Throat Chakra
Color: Blue/lavender

Location: Base of the throat

Basic Description: Sometimes called by the Sanskrit name "Vishudda" ("purification"), the throat chakra serves as a passageway between the head and the lower parts of the human body. The primary function of this chakra is self-expression and the art of communication with others. This communication and self-expression generally happen through sound—the vibrations of which can be experienced in both auditory and bodily ways. Sound has the power to become an entire energetic experience

In Balance: When the Throat chakra is in balance, people will feel energetically empowered to speak their truth. An open throat chakra allows for honest and confident communication. The words coming out will be powerful, enlightened, authentic, and directed. People will be able to pour their truths upon the world like honey, liberating themselves in the process.

Out of Balance: Throat chakra imbalance may manifest psychologically as lying, being overly secretive, or living in extreme fear. It manifests physically as chronic sore throat, voice hoarseness, or other mouth or dental issues. Neck pain is, and headaches are another common symptom of imbalance, along with jaw disorders. Emotionally, an imbalanced throat chakra can elicit a general fear of speaking out and self-expression. It can lead to untrustworthiness and telling other people's secrets, as well as the inability to listen to other people. It is not uncommon to see a decrease in social skills and creativity and an increase in anxiety and detachment from other people.

Heart Chakra

Color: Green

Location: Chest center

Basic Description: Also known by the Sanskrit name "Anahata" (unstruck), the heart chakra is the center of compassion, beauty, and the transformative experience of love. This chakra seeks connection in the form of giving and receiving love to others and opening oneself in love. It relates to the human capacity to love, the transcendence of personal identity into true connection, perceptions of beauty, and the experience of meaningful relationships. This chakra is tied to the cardiac and respiratory systems, as well as to the immune system through its association with the thymus gland.

In Balance: When the Heart chakra is balanced, there will be an increase of empathy in people's relationships as they are able to truly relate to those around them and hold compassionate space for them. A balanced Heart chakra leads to increased self-love, self-acceptance, and self-forgiveness, which therefore makes it easier to offer these same gifts to others. True peace can be achieved through an increased ability to process grief and heal the places where the heart has hardened or broken in the past. Additionally, the sense of harmonious connection to other beings and the world will deepen.

Out of Balance: Psychologically, an imbalanced heart chakra may manifest as extreme jealousy, resistance to intimacy with others, isolation, a savior complex, or unhealthy codependency. On a physical level, imbalanced heart chakras may cause issues with the heart and circulatory system, or increase risks for respiratory diseases such as bronchitis and pneumonia. Emotionally, a person with an imbalanced Heart chakra will have a much harder time forgiving themselves and others. They will also be more likely to put up walls and practice potentially harmful defense mechanisms and will be quick to shut down and fall into the role of the victim.

Solar Plexus Chakra
Color: Yellow

Location: Stomach/abdomen

Basic Description: Also called by the Sanskrit name "Manipura" ("city of jewels"), the Solar Plexus chakra is known as the energy center which embodies the most personal power. This center is all about personal abilities, willpower, and powerful assertion within the world. This chakra relates to the prospect of taking responsibility and control over one's own life and destiny with clarity, confidence, self-discipline, intellect, and self-awareness. This chakra is known for its expression of life purpose and larger plans.

In Balance: When the Solar Plexus Chakra is balanced, people will be more assertive in achieving the results they want and need. Their orientation in the world will be harmonious, and they will be able to maintain the energy necessary to get where they want to go.

Out of Balance: Imbalances in the Solar Plexus chakra can manifest psychologically as control issues, obsessive disorders, and the tendency to become manipulative over other people. Emotionally, imbalance of the Solar Plexus chakra may cause feelings of helplessness and lack of a clear life purpose. It can also lead to a lack of follow through on tasks, plans, and relationships.

Sacral Chakra

Color: Orange

Location: Below the navel

Basic Description: Commonly called by the Sanskrit name 'Svadhisthana" ("your own place"), the Sacral chakra is tied to the emotions, body, sensuality, and sense of playful creativity and fantasy. It plays an important role in sensations, the emotional experience, and the ability for people to truly be present in both their inner and outer worlds. This chakra plays an important role in relationship building and has a special role to play when it comes to sensuality, pleasure, and sexuality. The primary motivation of this chakra is pleasure, and pleasurable experiences are what motivate a general sense of well-being and openness to the world. This chakra connects to the genital areas, as well as the lymphatic system.

In Balance: A balanced Sacral chakra creates a harmonious and pleasurable state of being in relation to other people and the world. This relationship is centered around nurturing others and sharing pleasure with them, and it allows for human beings to expand and create their identities.

Out of Balance: Psychologically, an out of balance Sacral chakra can lead to emotional numbness and deep disconnection with oneself and their emotional experience. Dependency and addictive behaviors are common due to the desire to access pleasure. Physically, imbalance in the Sacral chakra can cause a lack of sexual desire, dissatisfaction, or sexual dysfunction. On an emotional level, an imbalanced Sacral chakra can lead a person to be overcome by their emotions to a point that is not functional. They may become stuck in particular emotional states and have a very hard time moving past them.

Root Chakra
Color: Red

Location: Base of the spine

Basic Description: Sometimes called by the Sanskrit name "Muladhara" ("foundation"), the Root chakra is associated with grounding and laying a foundation for the rest of a person's life. It is tied to feelings of security, self-preservation, meeting basic needs, and being physically present in the body. The Root chakra grounds people to the earth and helps to channel their energy into practical and self-preserving ways that aid survival and safety.

In Balance: The Root chakra is the space on which people begin to construct their lives. When it is balanced, it provides constant growth, positive orientation in the world, and feeling safe enough to explore all life has to offer.

Out of Balance: Psychologically, an imbalanced Root chakra may lead to disordered eating, cynicism, and living in a constant state of fight or flight mode. People with imbalanced Root chakras are likely to suffer from severe anxiety over the idea that they can never be fully secure. Emotionally, a person with an imbalanced Root chakra is likely to be more negative, insecure with themselves in the world around them, greedy, and covetous. People with imbalanced Root chakras likely feel far more threatened in the world and may have trouble being able to obtain feelings of peace and safety.

Chapter 5: Bringing Yourself into Balance

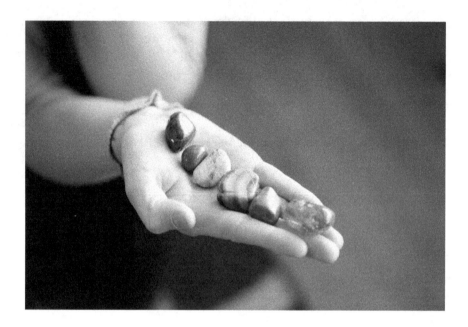

Crystals and Corresponding Chakras

The healing power of crystals has been harnessed for centuries to strengthen and balance the chakras. If you need a place to start, here is a guide of which crystals pair well with each chakra and why.

Root Chakra: If your root chakra is out of balance, you will likely be struggling with a lack of stability, feelings of insecurity, very limited willpower, and a general inability to become grounded. **_Smoky quartz_** has strong balancing properties that can be used to harness energy and increase protection and grounding. **_Zircon_** increases balance, as well as the ability to sustain it and reach high levels of purity and unity with all that is. **Hematite** is another great stone for balancing the Root chakra and becoming grounded because it balances yin/yang. **Black Obsidian** also helps with grounding, as well as increasing levels of security and aiding in a person's ability to be introspective. **Black Tourmaline** is a stone that helps ward off negativity and increases vitality. Garnet is another energy-increasing stone, which also aids in the establishment of stronger willpower, devotion, and commitment to obtaining balance and getting things done. **Red Zincite** is one of the rarest stones which aligns with the Root chakra, and it aids in the establishment of personal power and creativity. This stone is also very effective at removing energy blockages and rejuvenating the body.

Sacral Chakra: If the Sacral Chakra is out of balance, people may experience a lack of creativity, reduced sexual desire and satisfaction, infertility, extreme disconnection from intuition and emotionality, and a general sense of unwellness. **Vanadinite** is a stone that allows people to enter an elevated mental state, such as in meditation, wherein a person can reach a deeper understanding and restore a sense of order to their life. *Tourmaline* can be utilized in both blue and green forms to balance the sacral chakra. **Green Tourmaline** aids creative processes, life abundance, and the healing process. **Blue Tourmaline** facilitates effective communication and increased life awareness. **Carnelian** can be used to bring things back into balance by increasing perception and warding off negativity in daily life. **Imperial Topaz** is another option for balancing the Sacral Chakra, as it promotes deep creativity, the freedom of self-expression, and the restoration of energy and love. **Orange Calcite** is a stone with properties that can open and clear out all chakra centers, allowing for increased energy and overall healing.

Solar Plexus Chakra: When the Solar Plexus Chakra is imbalanced, people are likely to be lethargic, uninspired, lacking ambition, and generally lacking a sense of personal power. **Gold Tiger Eye** works to restore optimism, awareness, and life balance. **Golden Calcite** is a stone that can be used to drastically increase energy levels and corresponding ambition. **Yellow Apatite** works to stimulate the self-realization necessary for change. **Citrine** is one of the most powerful stones for clearing negative energies, building endurance, promoting enthusiasm, and expanding levels of self-esteem and life abundance.

Heart Chakra: When the heart chakra is out of balance, people will struggle more with being compassionate and extending love towards others. They may lack the ability to balance emotions and may also be far removed from consciousness. There are three types of Tourmaline that aid in balancing the Heart Chakra. The first is **Rubellite (dark pink) Tourmaline,** which restores creativity and loving devotion. **Pink Tourmaline** also aids in love, as well as increased understanding, spirituality, sense of calm, and capacity for joy. **Watermelon Tourmaline** works similarly as it specifically activates the energy of the Heart Chakra and helps clear blockages. **Lepidolite** restores honesty and helps create feelings of hope in the midst of life challenges and relationship difficulties. **Green Aventurine** aids in the balance of male and female energies, which can be incredibly helpful in creating balance in relationships. **Pink Danburite** is a purifying stone that aids in the removal of toxins from the body and helps restore communication and relationship building. **Malachite** is a necessary stone for the power of transformation, which is required to fully balance the Heart Chakra. This stone helps people grow in understanding and compassion of their own body and life experience and increases personal power and intuition. It may lead people to become more aware of how emotions are manifested physically in their bodies and take responsibility to make the changes needed. **Rose Quartz**, the stone of love itself, is the most powerful stone for balancing the Heart Chakra. This stone helps replace negative energy in relationships with positive energy, emotional harmony, compassion, and sexual balance. This stone also aids in forgiveness of the past and helps release negative emotions that are stored (like anger, fear, and jealousy).

Throat Chakra: If the Throat Chakra is imbalanced, people will face greater barriers to communication and self-expression, and are likely to lack a strong sense of purpose. **Aquamarine** is known for inspiring the courage necessary to look inside oneself and become truly aware of the areas which are lacking. **Celestite** is helpful in developing communication skills, fostering harmony, and clearing the mind. **Chrysocolla** aids communication as well by providing people with a more profound inner strength. **Amazonite** can be used to soothe a person into a place where they feel safer to open up and can more easily become attuned to spirituality. **Blue Kyanite** is useful for fostering the mental awareness necessary for effective communication. **Sodalite** aids in truth-telling. **Blue Chalcedony** helps balance energies of the body, mind, and spirit, and is widely used for improving group dynamics and kind, harmonious communication.

Third Eye Chakra: When the Third Eye Chakra is out of balance, people are likely to lack spiritual attunement and intuition. As the "Stone of Heaven," **Azurite** is known for stimulating the Third Eye in deeper intuition, sense of Enlightenment, and even psychic abilities. **Tanzanite** is a stone which yields cohesivity of personal power, psychic power, and the spiritual realm. Additionally, this stone can be a source of guidance on a person's journey to self-actualization.

Crown Chakra: Imbalanced Crown Chakras produce difficulty in obtaining higher consciousness. **Selenite** grants the mental clarity necessary to gain deeper insight and awareness, sometimes even into past and future lives. **White Topaz** is useful in stimulating energy, a sense of individuality, and thought patterns and loving actions that lead people towards their highest selves. **White Howlite** can serve to eliminate the negative emotions of stress, anger, and physical or emotional pain, while also increasing discernment and personal progress. **White Danburite** helps with increased intellectualism. **Amethyst** has the ability to abolish illusions about the world and aid in channeling abilities. This stone is known for producing greater peace, contentment, and personal strength. As the "Crystal of Attunement," the **Herkimer Diamond** can develop a sense of harmony, awareness, and a deeper connection to all that is. **Apophyllite** is the stone that bridges the gap between the physical and spiritual realms, facilitating astral travel, future gazing, and a sense of universal love and purity.

Plants, Herbs, Oils, and Corresponding Chakras

Root Chakra: The Root Chakra is responsible for keeping us grounded not only to the physical earth but also in the present moment. **Dandelion root** can be used to treat out of balance Root Chakras and work to heal depression, autoimmune diseases, low immunity, and pain in the lower parts of the body (legs, feet, tailbone, etc.) Consuming **root vegetables**, such as garlic, onions, carrots, and potatoes, can also be healing to the Root Chakra.

Sacral Chakra: When the Sacral Chakra is out of balance, the aromatic **gardenia** can be used for its roots or oil to restore creativity and happiness. There are a number of **herbs and spices** which aid in restoring the Sacral Chakra to full creativity, sensuality, and self-expression, including cinnamon, vanilla, Coriander, licorice, and fennel. **Sandalwood** can be applied to the body in oil form or burned in herb form to unblock the Sacral Chakra and aid in fertility, recovery from disordered eating, curing infection, protecting the urinary tract, and overcoming emotional imbalances.

Solar Plexus Chakra: Several **herbs and spices** used to facilitate emotional wellbeing and self-control include: peppermint, ginger, Lily of the valley, cinnamon, turmeric, and cumin. **Bergamot** can be used (most commonly in oil form) to aid in digestive health.

Lavender oil can be used on the body or diffused in the air or a bath to bring people out of depressed, anxious, or untrusting states of being into a state of calm mental and bodily relaxation. This is incredibly important, because poor mental health, self-doubt, and feelings of unworthiness can lead to digestive issues, liver and kidney issues, eating disorders, and ulcers. **Rosemary** is used in oil or herb form to calm the stomach and restore intestinal health.

Heart Chakra: **Hawthorne berries** in a tincture or a tea are one of the best herbal remedies for healing the heart chakra from grief, anger, jealousy, loneliness, hatred, and difficulty loving ourselves and others. By resolving these emotional issues, our sense of empathy, spiritual devotion, and physical hearth health and circulation can be restored. Several other useful **oils and herbs** for balancing the Heart Chakra are: rose, lavender, thyme, basil, jasmine, sage, cilantro, and Cayenne.

Throat Chakra: The issues with self-expression and difficulty communicating that arise with a blocked Throat Chakra can be aided by the use of **red clover blossom**, typically in the form of a tea. Healing of the Throat Chakra also aids in protection or recovery from issues with emotional codependence, spiritual insecurity, chronic fear, and anxiety, as well as physical issues with the thyroid or laryngitis. **Lemon balm** and **eucalyptus oil** applied topically to the chest are useful for thyroid health and throat decongestion. Several helpful **herbs and spices** for the throat chakra are lemongrass, sage, salt, and peppermint.

Third-Eye Chakra: **Mint** is a useful herb for healing depression by facilitating a deeper connection between the mind, body, and universe as a whole. It is also used to treat chronic migraines and improve memory and vigilance. **Eyebright** is an herb used to bring understanding of the "lights and darks" of life, produce a sense of mental clarity, and improve physical eye health. Juniper, jasmine, lavender, rosemary, and poppy seed are all useful *herbs and oils* for restoring imagination, intuition, and better sleep.

Crown Chakra: **Lotus flowers** are known to enhance a sense of divine wisdom and interconnectedness and restore a sense of universal connection in healing the Crown Chakra. **Lavender flowers** are also useful for enhancing meditation, bringing the soul into alignment, restring spiritual connection, and a sense of cosmic love. Teas, baths, aromatherapy, and some Japanese and Chinese dishes, are excellent ways to incorporate these flowers for healing.

Chakra Balancing Activities

Root Chakra: In order to balance the Root Chakra, your focus should be on grounding and coming back to connection with the earth. This can happen through any *outdoor activity.* Whether it's going for a hike, taking a walk, or simply finding a place in nature to sit, time in nature is crucial for bringing the Root Chakra into balance. *Grounding* is another effective practice for balancing the Root Chakra. This simply involves standing in the grass or soil with bare feet, preferably for a minimum of thirty minutes. In this time, the body can become saturated with the energies of the earth and fall back into balance with the rhythm of nature. If you can find at least fifteen minutes a day to stand with your bare feet on the earth, you are sure to notice a deeper sense of balance and presence in your environment.

Sacral Chakra: **Self-care practices** are vital for balancing the Sacral Chakra. This can come in the form of pampering oneself with a massage or a facial, taking a relaxing bubble bath, settling down with your favorite beverage and a good book, etc. Whatever self-care looks like for you, your Sacral Chakra needs it. Allowing yourself to **become aware of your emotions** through journaling, art, listening to music, or watching a movie that stirs your emotions, is another important element to balancing the sacral chakra. **Dancing** is another excellent way to channel this emotional energy, especially improvisational/lyrical dance, which focuses on free-flowing movements. Another tip for balancing the Sacral Chakra is to **imagine yourself as a body of water**, whether this be in meditation while dancing or creating, or while swimming and becoming a part of the body of water you're emerged in.

Solar Plexus Chakra: **Exercise** is one of the best ways to balance the Solar Plexus chakra. This may be swimming, going for a run, going to the gym, or simply doing a few yoga poses or sit-ups. **Spending time in the sun** in the hours of the early morning (before 10 a.m.) or the evening (after 4 p.m.) is another great option for balancing the Solar Plexus Chakra and recharging your life center. Another great option for stimulating your life center and balancing the energies of the Solar Plexus Chakra is in **trying a new activity or visiting a new place.**

Heart Chakra: **Random acts of kindness/love** are the best way to restore and balance your Heart Chakra. Doing kind things for other people helps your heart to soften, open, and generate loving energy in the world. **Connecting deeply with other people** through shared

74

smiles, eye contact, and intense "heart-to-heart" conversations are another excellent way to get energy flowing in your Heart Chakra. Another way to restore balance, especially when the Heart Chakra feels particularly hardened, tense, angry, or emotionally blocked off, is to come back to the moment with **deep breathing**. Breathe love in, and exhale anxiety, anger, hatred, fear.

Throat Chakra: **Writing** is a great way to put your truth into words, coming to terms with your own voice and experience and restoring the balance and self-expression to the Throat Chakra. If you find yourself struggling to share your truth verbally, writing is one of the best ways to get you back to that space. When you are ready, another way to balance the Throat Chakra is by allowing yourself to **share your voice** in conversations, not holding back on your thoughts and feelings. Remind yourself as many times as you need to that what you have to say is valid and worth being embraced.

Third-Eye Chakra: Your intuition and feelings of deeper purpose are achieved by **turning inward**. **Visualization practices** are crucial for restoring balance to the Third Eye Chakra. This may look like imagining yourself reaching your goals, achieving what you dream of, or being in a scenario where you are entirely at peace. This can also be allowing yourself to **imagine your highest self**. How does your highest self orient in the world? What is important to them? Which elements of their personality are most prominent? What is their lifestyle?

Crown Chakra: **Meditation** is the key to a balanced Crown Chakra. It is important to find some way to meditate every single day, even if it is only for 1-5 minutes. It is during this time that you can cultivate the silence, awareness, and openness that is required to feel fully in touch with your highest self. Allow yourself *quiet time* every day, *without distraction*, to have this experience.

Chapter 6: Chakra Check-In

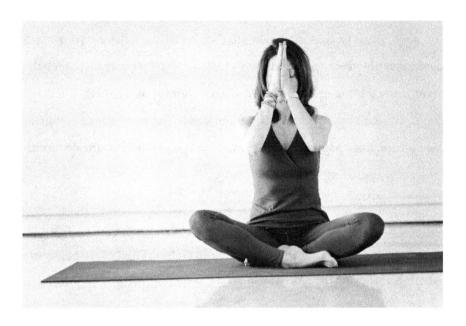

Daily Energy Check-in to Monitor your Chakras

The following practice is derived from the energy healing practice of *reiki,* which involves restoring balance to each of the body's energy centers through touch/hands-on healing. While most reiki practice requires certification, this technique is one that you can do on yourself daily without any formal training.

In this practice, you will be laying your hands on various parts of your body. Begin by washing your hands; you may apply a lightly-scented lotion or essential oil if it is pleasing to you.

Position 1- Hands Over Eyes: Place the palms of your hands over your eye sockets, with your fingers stretched up towards the top of your head.

Press lightly, holding for at least one minute. You may switch the position of your hands to have your fingers pointing inwards towards your nose, or outwards in a triangular shape to the sides of your head. Regardless of which position you choose, allow yourself to feel the movement of your eyes. Relax your face, letting all tension fall away. Take notice of any sensations. One minute is the minimum amount of time to hold, but you may hold as long as you want until you feel warmth in the area, and energy is freely flowing.

Position 2- Hands Over Ears: Cup your ears in your palms, gently clasping the back of your skull with your fingertips. You may massage lightly around the ears to ease any tension and drain lymphatic fluid. Remain here for at least one minute, holding as long as you need to feel the tension melt away and feel an increase of warm energy.

Position 3- Hands Over Temples: Move your hands to the sides of your head, clasping your thumbs underneath your jawbone. Press lightly into your temples, taking notice of any tingling, throbbing, or other sensations. Remain for at least one minute, or until you begin to feel the warmth or tingle of energy flow.

Position 4- Hands Over Whole Head: Place one hand horizontally across your forehead, clasping the crown of your head with the other hand. Press slightly harder, allowing yourself to come into the moment and feeling all distractions in your mind give way to clarity. This is one of the most grounding reiki positions, and you can use it on its own to center yourself throughout the day.

Position 5- Hands Over Throat: Clasp your hands around your throat in a crossed position (one over the other). Imagine your throat opening and your truth flowing freely from it. Take notice of any sensations you feel. You may also move your fingers to the side of your neck, keeping your palms centered, and begin to gently massage lymphatic fluid downwards towards the heart.

Position 6- Hands Over Heart: Position your fingertips towards the center of the chest, with your palms pressing just slightly above the nipple line. Feel the warmth and energy flowing into your chest, pulling slightly to the sides in an effort to "open" the heart. You may switch positions, moving your fingertips to face the navel. Hold for at least one minute, observing any sensation that arises as your heart opens.

Position 7- Hands Over Abdomen: Place your hands about midway down your torso, slightly above your navel. Point your fingertips inwards towards each other. Hold yourself securely, imagining restoration of your life force. Feel any weightiness or other sensations that arise in your stomach area. Hold for at least one minute.

Position 8- Hands Over Sacrum: Angle your fingertips down slightly, creating a triangular shape around your hips/lower abdomen. Notice any sensations of tingling, arousal, etc. that arise. Hold the energy here for at least one minute, warming and opening.

Position 9- Hands Over Thighs: To balance the Root Chakra, place your palms on the tops of your thighs, fingertips pointing downwards. Hold for at least one minute, allowing yourself to feel grounded up through your spine and down through the soles of your feet.

Chakra Check-In Daily Meditation With Journaling (Week 4)

After completing your basic chakra check-in, grab a pen and some paper and write out each of the seven chakras with some space next to it (Crown, Third Eye, Throat, Heart, Solar Plexus, Sacral, Root)

Consider each chakra, one by one, with the question, "What do I observe in my *particular chakra* today?"

Write down your levels of balance and any feelings you have about the energy in each chakra

Consider the chakras which feel most out of balance and ask yourself, "What am I going to integrate into my life today to re-balance these chakras?" Write your ideas down.

PART III

Section 3: Energy Healing

The Role of Energy in Holistic Health and Healing

Chapter 1: Energy Healing- The Key to Holistic Health

Understanding the impacts of energy imbalances and corresponding physical, mental, spiritual health

How many times have you, or another adult in your life, said the words "I just don't have the energy I used to have."? Most adults know the feeling of looking at the energy children have as they run about, enjoying life, exploring their surroundings, and never seeming to grow tired. Many of us are left reflecting back on the distant past when we, too, had such energy and wondering where it went.

From the time children enter school, they begin to be presented with expectations. Stand in a straight line, raise your hand, don't talk while the teacher is talking. Each year, the level of responsibility and expectation seems to increase. While rules, regulations, and individual responsibility are important for a functioning society, there are numerous expectations and social pressures put on people as they grow, which can be incredibly harmful.

It is generally around middle school when children become more acutely aware of their bodies and societal beauty standards, which tell them what they "should" look like. Children are likely to become aware of the trends, such as which clothes the "cool kids" are wearing. The endless battle to feel like enough begins, and can lead to a plethora of issues with self-esteem, eating disorders, and mental illness. In addition to the basic societal pressures to be accepted and considered attractive, many children are also faced with difficult situations at home where their own needs are not being met, they are having to provide for and protect themselves in the only ways they know how, avoid abusive parents, care for younger siblings, or worry about if they'll have anything to eat that day. Even if children have a relatively healthy home life, this is the age when they will begin to become aware of the issues that plague their family (every family has issues) whether this is divorce, an alcoholic parent, the death of a pet or loved one, etc.

We live in a society that thrives off of consumerism. We are flooded with images of how the next vacation, new pair of shoes, nicer car, nicer house, or perfect partner will make us happy, and all of the things we need to change about ourselves in order to fulfill those things. Eventually, all the energy we had as a child starts going towards maintaining our image in society, trying to have all the "best" life has to offer (which always happens to be everything we do not have), and attempting to be as "successful" as possible in the eyes of society and other people. With no time to rest in the present moment, recharge, and appreciate what we already have, it is no wonder, so many of us are completely drained of energy. In such a fast-paced society that discourages breaks, our energy will become depleted, and we will find ourselves thrown out of balance and unable to obtain true happiness and well-being. Over time, this depletion and imbalance can lead to a sense of spiritual disconnection, extreme mental health issues, and an increased risk of physical pain, illness, and even earlier death.

Chapter 2: Energy Healing and Overcoming Suffering

Energy and Grief/Trauma

Every human being knows that loss is a natural part of life. The one certain thing in life is that we, and everyone we know, is going to die. However, in such a fast-paced society, we are often given a very short grace period before being expected to swallow our grief and "move on" when we lose those closest to us. It is not abnormal for people to receive a bereavement period of only a few days before being expected to be back in the classroom or office and be fully functional. There is very little space for the grief journey, and most people are expected to harbor their feelings and keep their grief to themselves.

The grief process is expansive and incredibly energy draining. When we don't receive the adequate support from those around us, or adequate space to heal, our body begins to break down piece by piece. The empty spaces within us will swallow us up into states of depression, numbness, isolation, and pure exhaustion. Just like a wound being denied the correct treatment and care, the wounds of unresolved grief will fester and leave us feeling completely drained of energy and vitality for life.

Unresolved trauma also has an incredibly destructive impact on the body. Trauma can occur as a result of grief itself, as well as emotional or domestic abuse, accident or illness, war, sexual assault, childhood maltreatment, etc. The body holds trauma in various places, and the brain switches over from the logical ability to discern safety and danger into an easily triggered emotional state. An overactive emotional brain loses the ability to think clearly, make decisions, and recognize threats. People who have unresolved trauma are likely to be easily triggered and deal with unexplained outbursts of anger, fear, relationship issues, reckless behavior, and health problems. When trauma sits in the body unresolved, the brain is unable to understand that the traumatic event has ended. Therefore, it will stay in a consistent fight-or-flight state, which is incredibly draining and will leave the body with no energy. Not only will trauma victims experience low energy levels, but they will also experience severe issues maintaining positive relationships and overall well-being.

Energy and Mental Health

There are numerous factors that can contribute to mental health issues. As previously discussed, societal issues and unresolved grief and trauma can yield higher levels of anxiety, depression, and PTSD. It is also very common for people to suffer from mood disorders, personality disorders, disordered eating, substance abuse, etc. The list is long for psychological ailments and how they happen, and it has been proven that 1 in 3 people will be diagnosed with a mental illness in their lifetime. Even without a specific disorder, most people will have periods of life where their mental health suffers greatly.

No matter what a person's struggle with mental health looks like, or what they are doing (or not doing) in terms of treatment, the body expends a lot of energy when a part of it is unwell.

Daily Energy Regulation

No matter what it is in your life that is causing you to feel depleted, it is vital to pay attention to the energy fields within the body and identify the areas of greatest pain and imbalance. In the spectrum of health, people often take measures such as going to see the doctor, therapist, or grief counselor, taking medication, and making lifestyle changes such as finding a hobby or increasing exercise. However, a piece that is commonly overlooked in the healing journey is healing energetically. No matter how much you invest in your mental, physical, emotional, and spiritual health, if your energies remain imbalanced, it is impossible to reach a state of full wellness. That being said, energy healing is the missing piece in most people's quests for holistic health.

In many cases, it can be beneficial to seek the help of energy healers, massage therapists, and reiki, craniosacral therapy, or bodywork practitioners. These practitioners are trained in getting in touch with your energy centers and helping bring them back into balance through healing touch, body movements, and visualization techniques. If you are dealing with energy imbalance, seeing a practitioner can be an excellent investment in unlocking your highest levels of health and joy in life.

It is also possible to use a variation of the body scan mediation from chapter 3 to check in with your energy levels on your own. By taking notice of the sensations in each area of your body, you can come closer in touch with any area of your body where you experience regular pain, tension, or other unpleasant feelings. This is often a sign of imbalance or trapped energy. Additionally, the tense and release technique in each area of the body can yield healing and balance by releasing negative energy and tension. It is important to check in with yourself daily, asking your body where energy may be trapped or depleted and what you can do to replenish yourself.

Chapter 3: The Daily Energy Healing Journey

Understanding Your Energy Field: Daily Energy Healing Meditation with Journaling (Week 5)

There is a great variety when it comes to human energy fields. People experience varying levels of sensitivity to the energy of other people and the environment. Some people are incredibly in tune with "vibes"; others are empaths who feel the emotional experiences of others on a deep level, while still others experience very little of either. There is also a lot of variation in the way people recharge energetically, as well as what depletes them. In the common case of introverts and extroverts, for example, introverts need time alone to replenish their energy and feel balanced, while extroverts recharge in stimulating environments with other people around. One of the first steps to protecting your personal energetic field is to understand how it works.

Understanding Your Energy Field Journal Prompt (Week 5):

When you feel exhausted and not like yourself, which activities are most likely to replenish your energy? Do you enjoy a night out with friends? Yoga? A walk in the park? Leisure reading? Finding a new adventure? Taking a bubble bath? Listening to your favorite music on blast? List 5-10 activities that help you gain balance and feel energized.

Now, make a list of the things that make you feel most drained. These can be large things, like a specific task at your job, or small things like doing the dishes. You may find that you feel drained if you spend too much time alone or, consequently, when you spend too much time around other people.

When it comes to activities that make you feel drained, ask yourself to what extent that specific thing is necessary in your life. If you find yourself feeling drained from spending too much time around other people, for example, you can easily make a change by scheduling more "nothing time" or "alone time" into your days and taking the time you need to replenish. Household tasks and daily responsibilities are necessary, but by being aware of the ones that drain you the most, you can bring more attention to the process and doing what you need to replenish energy before or after.

Protecting Your Energy Field: Daily Energy Healing Meditation with Journaling (Week 6)

Close your eyes and ask yourself, "what does my energy field look like?" Write down any specific colors, textures, shapes, or patterns of movement.

Once you have an image in your mind of your energy field, ask yourself, "What does it look like for outside energies to enter my field?" Write down what healthy and unhealthy outside energies look like.

Then ask yourself, "How can I regulate the energies entering my field? What does it look like when I decide what I will let in?" Describe this process.

Finally, ask yourself, "How does my body feel when I regulate what I allow to enter my energy field?" Write down everything that comes to mind.

Healing Through Trapped Emotion Release: Daily Energy Healing Meditation with Journaling (Week 7)

In our society, we are often faced with life circumstances that force us to repress our basic human emotions. It is very possible for anger, rage, or grief to become stuck in the body because it is considered "impractical" to have those reactions in public. Similarly, we often hear about people being described as "annoyingly happy" or "overly emotional." Most of us are taught not only to manage our emotions but to distance ourselves from them and react emotionally only in certain contexts. Additionally, we tend to suppress negative emotions such as fear, shame, inadequacy, and insecurity, for the purpose of appearing like we have everything together. Between life events and societal expectations, it is very easy for the emotions we suppress to become trapped in our bodies, which can create adverse health effects, negatively impact our relationships, and keep us from living our best lives.

Begin by making a list of as many emotions as you can think of

Run down the list of emotions one by one, asking yourself, "Is there anywhere in my body I am holding *particular emotion*?"

Write down the emotions you feel are trapped. Take some time to journal about how certain emotions arose, or times when you felt you had to suppress your emotions.

With each emotion you have labeled as being trapped, write: "I give myself permission to release this *particular emotion*

Cultivating Self-Trust in your Healing Journey: Daily Energy Healing Meditation With Journaling (Week 8)

No matter what you do in your life, there will always be people who don't understand the choices you make, or who judge the path you are on. When it comes to renewing and protecting your energy, there is no room for anyone else's opinions or emotions in regards to your journey. It requires a great deal of self-trust to go your own way and let what other people think about it roll off your back. For this reason, it is vital to begin everyday establishing a sense of self-trust with your own journey and energy management skills. The following four journal questions will help you direct your energy before going about your day.

What are you most grateful for today?

What are your intentions for how you will direct your energy today?

What are your fears/things you perceive as a potential threat?

What are your commitments to yourself and the world?

One-Minute Energy Cleanse

- This meditation is useful if you find yourself with a person or in a specific situation that feels negative or energetically draining. You do not need to be alone to complete this meditation

- Pause where you are and allow yourself to take a few deep, cleansing breaths

- Focus exclusively on your breathing; you may close your eyes or leave them open

- Feel the inner power within the core of your body, around your abdomen. Remind yourself that you are in control and have the power to maintain balance.

- As you inhale, pull love, light, and peace into your body

- As you exhale, breathe out pain, annoyance, and toxicity

Energy from the Earth

- Begin by entering a space in nature. This can be on the beach, in the mountains, near a river, in a garden, by the lake, or in your own yard

- If possible, slip your shoes off, so your bare feet are in contact with the earth

- Start with a few cleansing breaths, taking note of everything you see, hear, smell, and feel in your environment

- Placing the soles of your feet on the ground, begin to breathe, pulling the energy from the earth up through your body

- Remember that you are One with the nature that courses around you. Allow it to heal what is broken within you and leave you feeling rejuvenated

Re-Centering Head Hold (3-5 minute meditation)

- Close your eyes and place the palm of one hand horizontally across the crown of your head, and the other palm across your forehead (over the energetic points of the Crown and Third Eye chakras). This position can be done while standing, sitting, or lying down.

- While clutching your head in this position, bring attention to any sensations in your body. What needs your attention most right now?

- Allow yourself to come back to the present moment, feeling grounded in your body and in your experience

- Breathe in awareness, focus, and comfort, exhaling anxiety and distraction

- When you open your eyes, notice how you feel grounded in your space

The Cloak of Protection

- This meditation is useful for energy protection before going out into the world, whether that is to work, the supermarket, an appointment, etc.

- Although you do not know what kinds of energies you may encounter, or which people may try to take your energy from you, remind yourself that you are in control of your own energy and that you have the capacity to protect yourself

- Close your eyes and imagine a dark-blue, almost black cloak made of a soft, thick material like a velvet night sky. The cloak is full-length with a hood to protect all of your chakras.

- Imagine a ray of light outlining the cloak in whatever color(s) feel most magical, protective, and authentic to who you are

- Set off into the world knowing that you are safe within yourself and your energy cloak and that you do not need to be afraid

De-Cluttering your Space

- When energy is lacking or out of balance, the spaces we live in are likely to reflect that imbalance with clutter and messiness. The more we feel like we "don't have our lives together," the more likely we are to have a messy desk, dishes piling up in the sink, laundry that still needs to be folded, or a car that has not been cleared of trash

- Such spaces do not allow for peace and mental clarity and can be even more draining to come back to after a long day

- Dedicate yourself to one area of your life to de-clutter. This can be your kitchen, your car, your bedroom, etc. Close your eyes before beginning and take a few deep, cleansing breaths to approach the task calmly

- Begin to address all of the clutter in the space, not only picking it up but putting it into a designated area where it can be organized and easy to find

- You may find that you want to create a special shelf or move some furniture around to make the space less cluttered. As you go, notice the energy that continues to unfold in your body

- When you finish, place a "clutter basket" in your room, the car, the living room, etc. where you can compile all the clutter throughout the day and put it away before bed

De-Cluttering your Mind (5-minute meditation)

- Close your eyes and begin to breathe deeply

- Ask yourself, "What is taking up the most space in my mind right now?"

- Bring your attention to whatever it is that is distracting you, and why it makes you feel out of control

- Breathe into that situation, saying, "I have control over this situation, and I am not going to let it spill out into the rest of my day. I am clearing this space."

The Energy-Ownership Mantra

- This meditation is ideal to perform in the morning, or before going out to interact with the world or other people

- Sit in a place where you feel energized (on the porch, in your meditation corner, etc.)

- Close your eyes and begin to breathe, checking in with any unresolved emotions or senses within the body

- Now begin to picture your energy field. Say to yourself: "My energy field is my sacred space, and other energies will only permeate it when I allow them to."

- Breathe into this thought for several moments

- Now, bring this thought into your mental space: "I have the wisdom to discern what belongs to me and what belongs to other people. I can be empathetic and attentive to other people's emotions, struggles, and opinions without assuming responsibility for them."

Epsom Bath Energy Renewal

- Begin by selecting your favorite scented Epsom salts. You may also customize your bath with petals, oils, and candles as according to the healing plants, herbs, and oils listed in Chapter 4

- Run a hot bath, letting your Epsom salts and other elements saturate the water

- Customize your space with the light of candles, meditative music, and anything else that makes you feel at peace

- Find a comfortable position inside the tub. Close your eyes, and feel your entire body relax into the heat and gentle movement of the water.

- Begin to conduct a body scan, feeling entirely vulnerable to this moment at peace with only yourself

- Ask your body, "What do I need right now?"

- The water should be hot enough that you begin to sweat (be sure to have a glass of water nearby). As you sweat, imagine your body purging itself of every blockage, every impurity, and every negativity

Sealing your Energy Field

- Close your eyes and begin to breathe

- Bring the image of your energy field to your mind. You may picture a wall, a bubble, or a glowing ring of light (this image may also differ depending on the day)

- Picture what other energies look like, floating around your field like particles in an atom. Say to yourself, "I am in control of what comes in."

- Imagine yourself recognizing people who are trying to take your energy or bear their burdens. Imagine any fear, anger, or resentment you may feel.

- Say to yourself, "No, not today." Imagine your bubble becoming impermeable, your wall being sealed, your glowing ring of light rejecting anything that does not belong inside
- Allow yourself to feel empowered over your energy, without feeling any resentment or judgment towards those who once posed a threat

Building your Sanctuary

- Sit down and close your eyes, beginning to breathe into yourself
- With each breath, ask yourself, "What makes me feel safe?" Repeat three times.
- Switch the phrase to "What makes me feel at peace?" Repeat three times.
- Switch the phrase to "What makes me feel loving?" Repeat three times
- Switch to "What makes me feel joy?"
- Lastly, ask yourself, "What makes me feel renewed?"
- When you ask yourself these questions, you may see certain crystals, scenes in nature, types of music, plants, aromas, decorations, activities, or color schemes. Take note of whatever comes to mind.
- Use these things that come to you in meditation to mindfully cultivate a space for yourself to come into every day when you need time to recharge. This can be a meditation corner, a spot

in the backyard, or any other space that is sacred to you and provides feelings of security and rest.

Cultivating Non-Reaction

- This meditation can be used when encountering a stressful situation, having a difficult conversation, or otherwise entering a state of nervous or angry energy

- Before responding to whatever the negative stimulant is, breathe into the moment. Close your eyes if needed.

- Tell yourself, "I can choose not to expend energy on this interaction. I can choose to move peacefully into the next moment."

- Feel the tension within you melt away as you make the choice not to internalize the stress of the situation or the negative energy coming at you

Boundary Setting

- Find a quiet place to sit and self-reflect. Breathe into the moment

- After you have settled into your breath, ask yourself, "What people, circumstances, or tasks drain my energy and leave me feeling agitated or exhausted?"

- Allow the answers to rise into your consciousness at will. Meditate on every name, every task, every circumstance which makes you feel tense and throws your energy out of balance.

- With each name, circumstance, and task, say to yourself, "This *person, place, thing* has no power over me. I can maintain my energy in spite of it."

- Next, ask yourself, "Where do I need to draw the line with this *person, place, thing*?"

- Listen to your intuition tell you what your boundaries should be. Perhaps, this looks like gently cutting off a toxic person, or limiting your interaction time with them. It could be quitting a job that is no longer good for you or asking for accommodations to make your environment more positive. It could be telling someone who expects you to bear their burdens that their energies are no longer your responsibility. Or, perhaps it is to establish a self-care activity to do directly after a draining task.

Trigger Awareness

- If your energy has ever been thrown out of balance by trauma, there are likely still factors of your environment that can strike at any time, causing your body to react in the same way it did at the time of the trauma.

- Breathe into the moment, asking yourself, "what elements of my environment cause me to lose control of my logic and feel afraid, helpless, irrational, in pain, or otherwise unbalanced or unhealthy energetically."

- These elements are called "triggers." Bring your awareness to these triggers, simply allowing them to be there without judgment.

- Say to yourself, "that moment in time is over. I can now release myself."

Energetic Tapping

- Begin by determining 3-5 affirmations or manifestations for the day ahead ("I manifest peace," "I am content," "I am present," "I manifest energy," "I am growing," "I manifest healing," "I manifest loving-kindness," etc.)

- Breathe deeply, pondering the affirmations/manifestations

- Choose your first manifestation/affirmation. With your index and middle fingers on both hands, begin tapping lightly on the crown of your head, repeating the manifestation or affirmation three times

- Move to the temples, tapping and saying the manifestation/affirmation three times

- Repeat at the inner corners of the brow bone

- Repeat just above the brow line

- Repeat at the top of the cheekbones

- Repeat below the ear lobes at the crest of the jawbone

- Repeat at the top of the chest

- Repeat on the left wrist, then switch to the right wrist

- Switch to the next affirmation/manifestation and go through the process again, staying in touch with your breath throughout

Listening to your Intuition

- Find a space where you feel completely comfortable and relaxed
- Begin to breathe deeply, coming into the present moment
- Ask yourself, "What does my inner self need me to know right now?"
- Keep breathing, holding space for whatever answer arises
- If necessary, you can ask follow-up questions to yourself, like "Is there any threat I need to be prepared to protect myself from?" or "How can I best love the world today?" Or "What do I need to do to take care of myself today?"
- Continue to breathe and hold space, trusting that your heart will guide you to make the correct decisions for yourself

Memory Reclamation (specifically for healing of trauma victims)

- Find a space where you feel totally safe and undisturbed. It is best to do this meditation on a day where you can invest in self-care and rest.

- Begin to breathe, telling yourself, "I am safe. I am safe. I am safe."

- Allow the memory of a particularly traumatic event to come to your mind. Continue to breathe, telling yourself, "I am safe."

- Pay attention to the details of that memory. What do you see? What do you hear? What do you feel?

- As the memory progresses, allow it to release its energetic hold on your body. Tell yourself, "That was then. This is now. I am safe."

- Feel the trauma release its hold on you, restoring itself to a basic memory of the past

Defining your Needs

- Sit in a peaceful place, breathing into the moment

- Bring attention to any pain or unrest within your body. Without judgment, allow it to be there, asking if there is anything you should learn from it.

- Generally, where there is pain or unrest, there is a need being left unmet. Ask yourself, "What is it that I need?"

- Allow your needs to arise into your consciousness ("I need a day off for my mental health," "I need a trip into nature," "I need a bath," "I need a warm, nourishing meal," "I need to go to sleep early," etc.)

- Breathe into each need, envisioning yourself meeting that particular need

- Ask yourself, "Is there anyone else I need to make aware of these needs?"

- Envision yourself having a calm conversation about your needs with your boss, your partner, your family, or a friend. Envision them, reacting gently and yourself feeling better understood and supported.

- Continue to breathe into your capacity to meet your energetic needs and make those needs known to others.

"Nothing Time"

- Set aside a minimum of one hour of time with absolutely nothing scheduled

- Sit down, breathing into the moment. Tell yourself, "this is my time. I have nowhere to be, nothing to do; I do not need to feel rushed."

- Allow your deepest intuition to guide your next step. Do whatever comes to mind first

- While you proceed with your "nothing time," allow your breath to guide every move

Discovering your Support System

- Bring your attention to the present moment, focusing on your breath
- Ask yourself, "Who of the people I know understands and embraces me for who I truly am?"
- Breathe with each name that comes up, allowing loving-kindness and appreciation for that person to flow through your body
- Ask yourself, "Who in my life encourages me to reach my full potential?
- Repeat the action of breathing with each name that arises
- Ask yourself, "Who in my life do I feel most at rest with?"
- Repeat the action of breathing with each name that arises
- Continue to breathe, saying to yourself, "These are my people. This is my support system. I will allow myself to lean on them when I need to."

Glowing Love-Energy

- Find a restful position and begin to breathe
- Imagine the aura of your energy field. How big is it? What color is it?
- Say to yourself, "I am pure love. I have room to love the entire universe and everything in it."
- Continue to repeat this phrase with every breath. Picture the aura expanding and glowing brighter

Jaguar Spirit Animal Protection

- Bring yourself into the present moment with deep breathing
- From the depth of your being, say, "I call on the spirit of the jaguar to protect me."
- Feel the reverberations of the jaguar's protection through your body, aiding you in repelling negative energy and toxicity
- Imagine a fierce, beautiful guard of your energy field, encircling you with fierce love and security

Energetic Breathing (1-3-minute meditation)

- Take some space away from your everyday life (in the bathroom, in the car, etc.) to just breathe
- Implement the 5-5-7 breathing technique
- With every breath in, say to yourself, "I breathe in pure energy."
- With every breath out, say to yourself, "I breathe out *exhaustion, *toxicity, *negativity, etc."
- Continue until you feel the tingle of pure energy coursing through your veins

Energetic Dancing/Movement

- Find a space where you can be alone and feel completely secure
- Play a song that stirs your soul and emotions, causing you to have a visceral reaction in the body each time you hear it

- As the song begins, close your eyes and deep breathe, maybe swaying back and forth slightly

- When you feel ready, release your body to move as it feels led. No choreography, no expectations, simply letting the movement of the moment lead your body into a state of pure surrender and release

- Surrender entirely to the moment, trusting your body to release any tension or trauma

- Give your body the space and freedom to heal, coming into energetic harmony

The Art of Saying "No"

- Close your eyes and begin to breathe deeply

- Begin to consider the things that drain your energy. Perhaps you have a tendency to overcommit or find yourself stuck in a relationship or circumstance that no longer serves you. Breathe with each of these places where you feel stuck

- Say to yourself "I have the power to say 'no.'"

- Imagine yourself having the necessary conversation, turning down the opportunity, or simply choosing to remove yourself from the situation

- Feel the power of saying no and being in full control of where you place your energy

The Restorative Power of Letting Go

- Breathe deeply, cultivating a sense of full peace and security
- Ask yourself, "Where are the parts of me that I need to get back?"
- Take notice of every person or place that comes to mind as still having a part of your energy and your essence
- If there are any feelings of melancholy, nostalgia, resentment, shame, or anger, allow them to be there, breathing as they flow through you
- Say to yourself, "I release this *person or place*. I reclaim what they have that is rightfully mine."
- Continue to breathe into this empowerment

PART IV

Chapter 1: The Empath

Imagine standing next to somebody on the street. You don't know them, nor have you have any type of communication with them. However, you can sense that this person is not doing well. They are sad and hurting on the inside. You don't understand why they have these feelings, but you know that they do because you can feel them within yourself too. This may sound like a far-fetched reality, but it's not. This is something that occurs when an individual is an empath.

Empathy means that you have the ability to sense and feel what someone is going through fully. This goes a step further than what we have already described in the first three chapters. While a highly sensitive person can understand and even relate to the emotions around them, an empath actually has the ability to feel those emotions within themselves. For example, if someone near an empath is sad and depressed, the empath will feel it inside of them as if they are standing in that person's shoes.

Dr. Judy Orloff, who is a professor of psychiatry at UCLA and a pioneer in the field of empathy, suggests that while highly sensitive people still have a barrier towards the stimulation in the environment, an empath has no filter, so absorbs everything around them like a sponge in a bowl of water. This makes it very hard for empaths to protect themselves and their emotions. They are also very sensitive sounds, strong personalities, and busy environments. They basically feel everything to a very high degree, and one of the reasons they become overwhelmed is because they cannot decipher or separate the emotions from their own. This means that as the emotions are coming in, like sadness, happiness, or anger, they have a hard time telling if they are feeling that way, or someone close to them is.

How To Tell If You're An Empath

There are many unique traits that empaths possess. The following are some of these qualities. If these sound familiar to you, then you may be an empath too.

- They are world-class nurturers and naturally giving. If you want someone by your side through thick and thin, then an empath is your person to go to.
- They are highly attuned to the environment around them, to the point that they feel everything down to their core. They might as well be standing inside of a person's body because they are feeling their emotions so closely.
- They are uncomfortable in large crowds because they are being inundated with all of the thoughts and feelings surrounding them, which can become very overwhelming and very exhausting.
- As a result of being uncomfortable in large crowds, empaths are often introverts. They usually prefer one-on-one interactions, rather than being in groups settings of any sort.
- Since it is draining for them to be around so many people, empaths need their alone time to help them recharge.

- They love nature as it nourishes and restores them. An empath would rather walk on a nice hiking trail than a city block.
- They have very finely tuned senses, so they are very sensitive to smells, noise, and excessive talking. If you touch an empath, don't be surprised if they jump a little bit.
- Since empaths can deeply feel the pain in others, they try very hard to relieve that pain for them, even if it's at their own expense.

The last person an empath thinks about is themselves. This is unfortunate because they are the ones who usually need the most care. While empaths have very appealing personalities on the surface, they often go through a lot of suffering because of the innate qualities they possess. The focus of this chapter will be the negative factors that come from having empathic traits.

Problems That Empaths Deal With

With all of the attributes that empaths have, they are bound to run into problems when dealing with the real world. While many people can separate themselves from others, it is nearly impossible for an empath to do the same. They are constantly sucked into the trials and tribulations of society, and as a result, are constantly dealing with significant emotional issues.

Empaths are often misunderstood. People who are not in their position cannot fathom what is going on in their minds. However, an empath is burdened with so many things that it becomes hard for their mind to cope with everything. If you know an empath or are one yourself, then you know exactly what I am talking about. The following are some of the challenges that these individuals have to deal with.

Their Feelings Can Be Flipped Easily

Imagine having the best day of your life. You are happy, energetic, and don't have a care in the world. You are on top of everything, and it seems that nothing can bring you down. Well, that is until something does. Of course, anyone of our moods can change quickly when something happens directly to us. This is not impossible. For an empath, though, nothing needs to happen to them directly. Once they are in the presence of someone who is emotionally distraught, their joyous mood can switch to a depressing mood instantly. Empaths are constantly shifting between various emotions due to the strong sensitivity they have with the environment. This puts them on a constant emotional rollercoaster. If they are in a group, the emotional fluctuations are even greater. From moment to moment, an empath will never know what his mood will be.

Emotional Fatigue Is Real

Dealing with our own emotions can be exhausting. Now, imagine adding several other people's emotions and having them be all over the spectrum. This can create heavy emotional fatigue.

Compassion Becomes A Burden

Empaths are often ridiculed for caring too much about other people. The truth is, it is hard for them to be any other way. They cannot turn off the compassion meter, which can become a burden after a while. Since an empath can feel suffering more than anyone else around them, it is difficult to not feel responsible for remedying it.

People Not Understanding Their Needs

Empaths are very likable, so people enjoy being around them. Many of them get invited out a lot. However, empaths need their alone time once in a while to recharge, but most people do not understand that. They believe they are just flaking on them, so they push them, even more, to go out. Unfortunately, most empaths will give in because they do not want to upset their friends.

Needing Time To Process Transitions

Empaths will have a hard time jumping from a high-stimulus to a low-stimulus environment. If they go from a crowded event to a small event, they will feel hollow for a while, trying to process the change. On the other hand, going into a suddenly crowded environment will overwhelm them.

It Can Be hard To Enjoy Yourself

Since you are always inundated with other people's feelings, it can be hard to enjoy yourself. You feel bad about feeling good, essentially, because you know that other people are suffering.

Get Taken Advantage Of

Because empaths care so much about other people, they often get taken advantage of. Certain types of people love to pounce on empaths because they know they can get away with a lot. We will talk more about these people later on.

Saying "No" Is Difficult

Empaths often feel guilty for saying "no," even though they need to say it more than anyone else. You are always willing to sacrifice your time and well-being for others until you hit a wall.

The struggles that empaths deal with are real. Unfortunately, their most unique qualities that are beneficial to other people have the most negative impact on them. Empaths must learn to use their characteristics in a way that helps others but does not overwhelm them. Otherwise, they will always live a life of suffrage.

What Creates An Empath

There is a wide range of reasons why a person becomes an empath. Some people are born with this mindset, while others develop it over time. This is the whole nature vs. nurture argument. Dr. Judy Orloff has described four different factors that contribute to empathy and becoming an empath.

- Some infants come out of the womb and are more sensitive to certain stimuli. For example, they cry more often and are extra sensitive to things like sound. Basically, people are born with different temperaments, which suggests that being an empath is a birthright to a degree.
- It is possible that there is a genetic component to being an empath. Many parents who are empaths often give birth to kids who are empaths too. However, this is not always the case, which means our genes are not the sole cause and may not have any connection in some cases.
- Children who are neglected or abused as a child often have their defenses torn down. They have experienced what it's like to be around a lack of sensitivity. In turn, they become extra sensitive as adults.
- Overly supportive parents can also create extra sensitive children. Children who take in many empath traits from their parents will carry them into adulthood.

Many researchers have found a significant amount of scientific backing related to being an empath. There is a specialized group of cells in our brains that are responsible for compassion. They enable everyone to mirror the emotions of the people close to them. These are known as mirror neurons, and they are thought to be hyper-responsive in empaths.

Empaths are also thought to have a stronger emotional contagion. This is a phenomenon where people can pick up on the emotions around them and then start feeling the same way. This can be seen in a room full of infants when one of them begins crying, and it sets off a cascade among the other babies too. Eventually, the whole room of infants is crying.

Finally, empaths are shown to have a higher sensitivity to dopamine, which is a neurotransmitter associated with the pleasure response. Dopamine is generally released when stimulated in some way. When an individual experiences a joyous moment, dopamine is released, which makes them even happier. Due to the higher sensitivity, empaths need less dopamine to increase their mood. This may explain why empaths are content being alone. They do not need a lot of external stimulation to feel good.

In summary, if you are an empath, then it is not something you can avoid. You are essentially stuck being an empath for the rest of your life. As you will see later on, this is not a bad thing. It is imperative, though, to manage the negative aspects of this quality, Which we will also get into more in the next couple of chapters.

Empaths And Toxic Relationships

While most people like empaths, the relationships they are in are not usually reciprocal. Meaning the compassion, kindness, and love that empaths give are not returned to them in the same manner. Of course, an empath would not expect these emotions to be displayed, but it's imperative to point out the lopsided relationships that many of them are involved in.

While many people take advantage of an empaths generosity, certain personality types take it to the extreme. These are the worst individuals for an empath to be around. They are collectively known as energy vampires and come in various forms. If you are an empath, you must recognize these energy suckers do that you can avoid them completely.

Energy vampires are the opposite of empaths. They lack any type of empathy, compassion, or emotional maturity, and do their best to take what they can from people. It is usually not through force, but with various manipulation tactics. Empaths, who are always willing to give, are the perfect victim for them. The following are different types of energy vampires that must be avoided.

The Victim

These vampires are always the martyr. They believe the world is out to get them and take no responsibility for their lives. They continually blame, manipulate, or blackmail to get what they want. The victim vampires feel unworthy in their lives, so they will work to garner sympathy by making you feel guilty.

The Narcissist

The Narcissist has no ability to show empathy and has no genuine interest in other people. They always expect to be put first, no matter the circumstances. They have giant egos that need to be fed, and they will always make sure not to go hungry. Narcissist vampires are dangerous because they will be very likable and charming at first to gain your trust, but then stab you in the back when it benefits them.

The Dominator

The dominator will make themselves feel superior through intimidation, whether physical or emotional. They are often loudmouths with rigid beliefs about how the world should be. Therefore, many of their viewpoints are archaic and can be seen as racist, sexist, or homophobic.

The Judgmental One

Judgmental vampire suffers from low self-worth. As a result, they project these feelings onto other people through shame and ridicule. Basically, they make themselves feel better by making you feel small.

The Innocent One

Unlike the other vampires, the innocent types are usually not malicious. They genuinely need help in their lives and are just looking for a hand. Their intent is not to harm anyone; they are just not emotionally strong enough to help themselves. That being said, you will still drain yourself if you are their constant rock to lean on. The key is to help but also to encourage self-sufficiency.

Unfortunately, many energy vampires are those who are closest to us, like family and lifelong friends. This makes it even easier to fall into their traps and get out energy sucked out by them. This makes it more imperative to be on high alert for their manipulative tactics.

The objective of this chapter was to paint a picture of what an empath is. Hopefully, you can visualize one in your mind. If you are an empath too, then you probably recognize many of the characteristics described here. Also, you have probably experienced the same setbacks. The remaining chapters in this book will focus on the positive aspects of being an empath and how you, as an empath, can share your gifts with the world, while also protecting yourself from harm.

Chapter 2: The Empath Blessing

In the previous chapter, I described in detail what an empath is and what challenges exist from being one. I admit that I probably did not paint the most appealing picture, but my goal was to make you aware of the specific empath traits so that you can recognize them within yourself and others. Once you do, then you can work on improving yourself by overcoming the obstacles that are in the way of your success.

The truth is, being an empath is a blessing because you bring so much value to the world. Some have described their abilities as paranormal, or as having a superpower. People rely on you because of the gifts you possess to be able to help them. The focus of this chapter will be to illustrate the positive impact that an empath can bring to those around them, in every facet of their lives. If you fall into this camp, just know that you are a very good addition to anyone's life.

Empaths As Leaders

Because of the unique personality traits an empath has, they are actually great leaders. They have a strong capability to create positive change within an organization. This is considering they don't allow themselves to be manipulated. The following are some of the top reasons that empaths can become successful leaders in any environment.

- They want to improve the world. Empaths are contributors, rather than takers, and want to improve human relationships by offering tremendous support.

- Empaths burden themselves with other people's issues, which may not be great in the long run, but can get a lot accomplished in real-time. Bearing this extra burden will often push empaths towards their goals.

- They have good relationship skills and can communicate better with those around them because of their deep understanding of the world.

- Their followers do not see them as intimidating, which means they are more willing to work with them.

- Empaths have a deep love for humanity, in general, so they do not discriminate against anybody.

- They look towards the future, not in the sense of making profits, but finding solutions that plague so many people.

- Even the most closed off and difficult people to work with will engage with an empath because they will provide a comfortable atmosphere to do so.

- They do not let success get to their heads, and they will not try to steal all the credit.

While empaths are not known for having strong personalities, they have endearing qualities that make them very likable and trustworthy. People are drawn to empaths, and this allows them to create successful teams with many different types of people. If empaths held more leadership roles, whether, in politics or business, the world might be a friendlier place.

Why Empaths Are Great Friends

Just like highly sensitive people, empaths have appealing personalities that make them great friends. As an empath yourself, just know that anyone is lucky to have you in their lives. Why do empaths make great friends? I will explain why.

Empaths Will Know When You're Not Well

Empaths will know stuff about you without you having to tell them. This is not in a creepy or intrusive way. They simply have the skills to pick up on various clues that you are unknowingly putting out. These abilities go beyond being intuitive and actually border on the paranormal. It is as if they can read your mind. As a result, an empath will know when you are upset, ill, tired, or going through any other negative emotion. There is no hiding your feelings when you are with an empath. Because they recognize the pain you are going through; they will have the compassion and understanding to help you get through it. If you have a problem, you can always count on your empath friend.

They Know The Right Things To Say

Because empaths are so good at picking up on the emotions of others, you rarely have to explain to them what you are going through. The chances are, they already know. This will save you a lot of pain and frustration, trying to explain what is wrong. Of course, if you want to explain it, an empath will listen with open ears.

When we are feeling negative, for whatever reason, it can be hard to get the point across to people because they are not going through our experiences. They are not living in our bodies. An empath will be by your side and will not ask unusual questions or completely miss the point about what you're saying. Finally, they will understand when to push forward with an issue and when to back off. In most cases, an empath will know what to say and the right time to say it.

They Can Protect You From Other People

There is something ironic to discuss here. Since empaths have such high compassion and kindness inside of them, they are willing to help almost anybody. On the other hand, an empath can help protect you from other toxic people. Because of their ability to understand people quickly, they can determine if a person is genuine or might have some ulterior motives. Therefore, if an empath has some unpleasant vibes about someone, it is in your best interest to listen.

Some people suggest not to be around anyone that an empath does not approve of. I will not go that far. However, never dismiss the feelings of an empath and always keep them in the back of your mind. Even if an individual seems perfect in every way, there might be some red flags you miss that an empath will recognize immediately. They will know if someone is dishonest and what their true intentions are. On that note, do not try to be dishonest with an empath because they will pick up on it quickly.

They Are Fun To Be Around

Being friends with an empath is an exciting experience because they are free spirits. They tend not to live in the norm and are always up for an adventure. If you're looking for a travel buddy, consider an empath because they are up for almost anything. You will have a blast. A word of caution: You may have to share your empath friend with other people because their personalities are attractive, even to strangers.

They Are Great Listeners

When you are speaking with an empath, you can be sure they are listening. They are not just listening so they can respond, but because they genuinely want to hear what you are saying. They will also help you come up with the best solutions since they understand you so well. However, if you are just talking to vent and are not looking for someone to solve your problems, an empath will understand that too and just listen without interrupting.

I want you to assess your current situation right now regarding your inner circle. Who are the types of people that you enjoy hanging out with the most? I want you to be completely honest with yourself. What personality traits do they carry? Do some of your best friends behave as empaths, at least partially? The chances are, those whom you genuinely enjoy being around possessed many of the innate attributes that are associated with empaths.

Seek out empath relationships, and you will not be disappointed. If you are an empath, then share your gifts with the world. Just make sure to keep yourself safe. I will discuss how to do this more in the next chapter.

The Empath As A Spouse

For the final showcasing of why being an empath is a blessing, I will discuss why empaths make great spouses. If you can find an empath as a partner, then you will be in a luckier place.

They Care About Making You Happy

With empaths, you do not have to worry about selfishness in a relationship. They want a happy life, and they understand that making their spouse happy is part of it. They are more concerned with having a genuine connection with their partners than they are with material possession.

They Make Amazing Parents

If you want children someday, then having an empath as a partner is a blessing because they make amazing parents. An issue that children deal with is that the adults in their lives don't understand them or pay attention to them. They often feel neglected and tossed aside. This will not be the case with an empath. They will be in tune with their children, just as much as they are with anyone else.

They Are Willing To Change For The Better

As a relationship grows, so must the people who are involved. Some individuals are so hardheaded that they are never willing to change. Empaths are so profoundly connected to the world and the people around them that they will recognize their shortcomings and will always be willing to work on them. If there are issues within a relationship, the empath will look inside of themselves and determine where they need to improve.

They Are More Tolerant And Understanding

Empaths understand that people are not perfect. They can also recognize the pain someone is experiencing on the inside. As a result, they are more patient, tolerant, and understanding of people's mistakes and shortcomings.

They Want You To Be Yourself

You do not have to put on a fake persona for an empath. They want you to be yourself. In fact, if you are trying to be fake, they will pick up on it quickly.

The Love Is Passionate

Empaths know how to make you happy. When they do make you happy, they will feel the same way. This will bring them a lot of joy and passion. The happier you are, the happier they will be. So, they will love you with great passion, and make you feel more accepted than anyone else can.

They Are Great At Working Through Disagreements

Since an empath can put themselves in your shoes, it is easier for them to see where you are coming from. They will be able to respond accordingly and work through disagreements more smoothly.

They Hold You Accountable

This may be one of the most important traits of being an empath. Since empaths really understand what you are going through, they will have compassion, but also know that you have the ability to fix it. As a result, they will hold you accountable for improving yourself and getting past whatever is harming you.

As you can see, an empath is a great leader, friend, partner, and pretty much anything else. As long as they are able to harness their power for the well-being of others while keeping themselves safe, they can do a lot of great things in this world. Don't be a stranger to an empath.

Chapter 3: Protecting Yourself

A knight in shining armor has the power to protect those who need him. However, without his armor, he will be harmed easily. The same holds true for an empath. An empath is a true blessing to the world, as we detailed in the previous chapter. However, without properly protecting themselves, an empath is at great risk for many negative consequences. Their mental and physical health, relationships, careers, and even personal safety can be affected, so they must take the proper precautions for their own well-being.

The focus of this final chapter will be about how an empath can protect themselves. I will go over some valuable tips and strategies to keep you safe so that you can continue to bless the world with your gifts. The reality is, once you burn out, you can no longer help others. This means that self-care is not just for you but also for the benefit of other people. The better you are to yourself, the better you can be to other people.

Protect Yourself Against Energy Vampires

While empaths can recognize a negative person because they are aware of people's true motivations, they still fall victim to toxic individuals. Their caring personalities can get the best of them, so they fall prey to people who use them the most. The obvious example here is energy vampires. These are any type of individuals who literally suck out your energy and make you feel drained. I described energy vampires in an earlier chapter, and now I will go over how to protect yourself as an empath from these energy stealers.

Realize They Exist

The first step in solving a problem is recognizing there is one. Energy vampires are a big problem for you if you are an empath. Empaths have a tendency to believe that all people are good and ignore the fact they are in a toxic relationship. Recall some of the characteristics I described for energy vampires and start realizing that bed people who want to take advantage of you do exist.

Keep A Journal Of Your Gut Instincts

Since empaths are highly intuitive, probably more so than anyone else, their gut instincts will tell them a lot about a person. As an empath, you must learn to listen to your gut instincts and never dismiss them, no matter how ridiculous they may seem at first. Also, after spending a lot of time with energy vampires, you can start losing the ability to believe how you feel. One thing these energy stealers are good at is manipulation.

When you are with someone, pay attention to what they are engaging in and write down how they make you feel inside. Pay special attention to how they treat a variety of people they encounter, like waitresses, flight attendants, and cashiers, etc. How an individual treats people who are not considered high on the status bar says a lot about who they are.

Have A Reality-Check Friend

A friend like this is an objective observer who has not been taken in by the energy vampire. They should be trustworthy and be able to their honest opinion about a person when your own judgment might be clouded.

Pat Yourself On The Back

Empaths often due not give themselves the credit they deserve, even though they are responsible for many of the good things around them. Instead, they deflect the credit onto someone else, effectively minimizing their own contributions. I don't want you to get a big head here, but I hope you can pat yourself on the back often recognize what you have accomplished. Write these accomplishments down on a piece of paper daily, so you have something visual to look at.

Put Yourself First

This should be the case no matter who you encounter in your life, but energy vampires are exceptionally good at making empaths feel guilty. They will use every manipulative tactic in existence to make sure they are at the forefront of your mind. They do not care about you unless you are doing something for them. So, make them stop caring. Whenever you feel like your in the presence of an energy vampire, take a step back. Leave the room completely if you have to. From here, remind yourself about your needs and that you deserve to live a joyful life. This will help keep you from falling into the vampire's trap.

Add "No" To Your Vocabulary

I don't care if you have to stand in front of the mirror all day repeating this word, but get as comfortable as you can saying the word "no." It is okay, and even necessary, to use this word once in a while. Empaths have a difficult time saying "no," and their knee-jerk reaction to anything is often "yes" without even considering their own feeling. I don't want you to automatically say "yes" to everything because you will not have the ability to set boundaries. If you have a hard time saying "no," at first, start with a lighter phrase like, let me think about it. Eventually, you can work yourself up as you feel comfortable. The main goal is t not be agreeable all the time.

Prioritize Your Own Quality Time

Set aside sometime every day for your own needs. Even if it is just 20 minutes, this time should be spent focused on your well-being and self-care. Do whatever makes you feel good at this moment, like meditation, reading, taking a bath, or going for a walk. Avoid things that might bring you stress, like social media drama, or watching the news. Stick to your guns about this self-care time, and do not let anyone interrupt it. Visualize all of your negative energy, disappearing into thin air.

Set Boundaries

Learn to set boundaries with people, or they will take up all of your time. As an empath, people will be vying for your attention because they know you will give it to them. You need to put the breaks on this mindset ASAP. I am not saying you can't help people. However, you need to put strict limits on how much time you will spend doing so, because you still need to fit in your self-care. If your friend needs help, set aside time when you can help them, but also place a strict time limit on the encounter. You cannot just be available any time of day for as long as they need it. This may sound insensitive, but it's really not. Your well-being is important too.

One of the ways to ensure you live a happy life as an empath is to keep toxic people away from you as much as they can. Vampires, like the many I have described, can sniff out the blood of an empath and dominate them into submission. If you are not careful, you will be under their control for the rest of your life. There may be times you cannot avoid toxic people; therefore, the techniques above can be used to distance yourself and avoid their tactics as much as you can.

Take regular stock of your friends too. The people in your inner circle should fill you up and make you feel good. If they are not doing that, then it's time to distance yourself or get rid of people completely. An energy vampire can infiltrate themselves into your life unsuspectedly. You must stay on high alert at all times for these individuals.

Harnessing Your Empath Power

Empaths have strengths that cannot be denied. The world needs these blessings now more than ever. This is why it's important to take care of your inner empath. We cannot afford to lose you. Once empaths learn how to harness their superpowers, they can become empath warriors and begin saving the world. Empaths who know how to save their energy are unstoppable because they know themselves well enough to practice self-care and stop absorbing the negative energy around them.

Going back to Dr. Judy Orloff, as an empath herself and someone who has researched the topic endlessly, she has come up with several strategies to harness your empath power and make you a true warrior in this respect. I encourage you to practice these techniques on a regular basis, so they become a habit for you.

- Express gratitude every day for what you have in life. Being grateful allows your mind to stay focused on positive energy by keeping you in the moment, rather than wasting energy worrying about the future.

- Practice different meditation techniques. There are many techniques out there that can help center you and make you in charge of your emotions. Mediation can take a while to master, but the initial goal is to reach a state of mindfulness

- Practice mindful breathing by focusing on your inhalation and exhalation. Breath in clarity and strength and breath out stress and negativity. Make sure you can feel your breaths down to your diaphragm. Practice these several times a day.

- Strengthen your intuition by learning to listen to it. Notice when your energy levels either increase or decrease when your around somebody. Stick with the people who make your energy levels go up.

- Practice loving yourself every day. Make sure to always engage in positive self-talk. How you speak to yourself plays a big role in your self-worth.

These exercises are simple and can start being used right away. When they become a regular part of your routine, you will be able to share your empath gifts, without being taken advantage of.

Best Careers For An Empath

To give yourself the best chance of winning, it is imperative to set up an environment that benefits you. You will never stop being an empath, and nor should that be your goal. However, it should be your goal to use your strengths in the best way possible. If you are like most people, then you need to work to make a living. It will behoove you to be in a setting that enhances your strengths and minimizes your weaknesses. The following are some of the best career options for empaths.

Nursing

Nursing would be a great career path for a naturally caring and compassionate person, like an empath. They will be using the skills they possess every day, providing the best care for people. Just be mindful that high-stress and fast-paced settings like the emergency room or the ICU can create some complications for the empath's psyche. However, this can be overcome with some practice and experience.

Artistic Careers

These include things like writing, painting, ceramics, or photography. Empaths are known to be creative individuals, so anything in this line of work will be great for them.

Psychologist Or Counselors

People in these careers need to be intuitive, kind, compassionate, and caring. They need to have a deep desire to help people and often have to read between the lines to get the real answers. An empath possesses all of these qualities, so they would excel in this career path.

Veterinarian

Empaths are not just great with people, but also animals. In fact, there is a subset of empaths who can relate to animals on a very deep level, almost as if they can read their thoughts and communicate with them. This is great since animals cannot speak for themselves. An empath who becomes a vet can help heal and comfort sick animals, and also soothe their worried owners.

Musician

Just like with an artist, an empath can let out their emotions and creativity in this line of work. There will also be opportunities to play so many different instruments, as well.

Teacher

There are very few people who need empathy in their lives more than children. Children cannot always express their needs with clarity, so having someone who understands them well is a huge plus. They will gravitate towards an empath because they feel comfortable around them. With proper motivation and support, a teacher could change a student's entire life.

As an empath, if you are looking for a career where you will thrive and none of the above interests you, that's okay. There are plenty of opportunities out there that will require your skillset. While you can succeed anywhere, jobs that require compassion, care, patience, intuitiveness, and kindness, while also being less fast-paced, might be the best pathways to take.

Being Kind To An Empath

I want to end this book by speaking to those on the opposite side. If you have gotten through this book and realized that you are not an empath, that's okay. The chances are that you know an empath, or will meet one at some point. I want to help you understand some important issues about being an empath so that you can bring the best out of them, and they can bring the best out of you. As I mentioned before, an empath will be one of the best people in your life, if you understand how the dynamics of the relationship will work. Here are a few important facts to remember.

- Empaths cannot change who they are. They can work on ways to protect themselves, so they are not used and abused, but they cannot stop being extra kind, compassionate, and caring.

- Empaths cannot be caged and become shut-ins. They have to get out and explore; otherwise, they will lose their zest for life.

- Empaths need time alone, so make sure they get it.

- They see life much differently than others, so give them support.

- They know if you're lying, so always be honest, even if it hurts.

- They love to laugh, so make them laugh often.

- They will be on an emotional rollercoaster, and so will you.

In summary, do not be with an empath if you can't handle life being different every day. If you can, then get ready for the time of your life.

PART V

Chapter 1: Anxiety, The Monster Within

"I know what it's like to be afraid of your own mind."

- Dr. Reid from Criminal Minds

- Obsessing over small worries that constantly distract you
- Whirling from action to action to try to quiet your minds' nagging
- Attempting to drown out anxious thoughts in any way possible, solemnly wishing they would just disappear

If you are here with us today, you are likely living through all the above and more, trying strategy after strategy to eliminate these causes of stress. Or, perhaps you are seeking help for a loved one that has anxiety that is weighing them down. Or, maybe you are simply here to feed your curiosity of what anxiety is and how it plagues the mind. No matter, I work with anxiety every day and have spent the majority of my existence on Earth immersed in it.

My grandfather was such a worrier that he physically shook, *constantly*. His body would tremble from the overwhelming magnitude of worry that lurked within him. He was a burly southern man who favored anything outdoors and fishing. His long, curly locks framed his rounded face with an always generous smile. When he was at his warmest, he was a magnet to others. However, his most natural state was when he was in worry mode.

What did he worry about? Anything and everything. He was worried about all the typical things that grandparents do; along with I'm sure many countless unspoken things.

"Do you have enough to eat?"

"Do you need the salt or pepper?"

"Are you comfortable? Too hot? Too cold?"

Even though he was a burly man, his voice was soft, so anyone listening had to lean in. I think he like the intimacy it afforded. Whenever we were all at ease, he was at ease.

Us grandkids always ran with the joke, *"Grampy, can we pass you the salt and pepper?"* His anxiousness would disappear with a smile and flush of embarrassment. We did this to show our appreciation, to relieve the tension and let him know he was never a burden and that we loved our big burly gramps for who he was.

Our gramps was a people-person, always curious and invested in others. I have very clear memories of coming home and hearing his low but small voice in the answering machine, *"Hello, it is just me again. Just checking in to see how you are coming along…"*

He needed that regular assurance that everything was, in fact, alright and always preferred to hear it firsthand. And if he could do things for someone, that was even better.

As Gramps aged, his anxiety escalated and he became less able to use it in a constructive manner. There were less and fewer ways for him to release his anxious feelings, to the point he became crippled with worried on a daily basis. When I search into where my own anxiety stemmed from, a picture of Grampy always pops into my mind. When I studied anxiety in graduate school, his shaking body was a perfect analogy. The more time I spent exposed to the study of anxiety in the human body, I began to understand my grandfather better than he likely understood himself most days. I also realized how persuasive anxiety was throughout our family's history. It was what set the foundation for me to deeply understand how much anxiety affected emotions and behaviors.

Thankfully, no one else in my family shook as much as my grandfather did from anxiety; however, looking back, anxiety was the hub of all the spectrum of extremes my family endured. My mother was motivated by her anxiety, while my father was like a balloon, letting stress and anxious feelings build up until he popped with rage.

While no one in my immediate family was ever diagnosed with an anxiety disorder, I can still imagine that just like so many others, they would have felt the same shameful stigma that comes along with all mental health problems, thinking that something is wrong with them. They were simply noticing things in their lives and felt deeply about them; they just didn't have the tools and knowledge to cope with the overload of information.

Through my years as a psychologist, I have gained a different perspective on anxiety and how it alters thoughts and feelings. I have come to see anxiety as a resource and seek to embrace its value in our everyday lives.

Anxiety derives from the feeling of realizing that something we genuinely care about may be at risk, as well as the arrival of resources that we need in order to protect it. Anxiety prompts us to look closer and pay better attention to messages we receive and helps us to gain the motivation we need to take control of situations. The key to getting back a life driven by anxiety and fear is to take control. This is where I have used my knowledge to help others, in ultimately steering them in a different direction of gaining back their willpower.

How Anxiety Overshadows Everyday Lives

Living in denial, second-guessing your every move, thinking ill thoughts about your future, living in fear of the unknown; all these things can overshadow a person's life and lead to constant anxiety.

If you or a loved one is plagued by anxiety, you have probably endured panic attacks and constant negative nagging in your head on a regular basis or have a phobia of some kind feel ashamed of their "sickness."

Anxiety has the power to make everyday folks feel insane, even though they truly aren't. Just like with all people, some days are better than others, but those who experience symptoms caused by these mental ailments typically have a higher count of bad than good days.

They often feel that they are always under a dark cloud that pours rain, but that rain is not made up of just water. Those drops from the sky above their head are created from startling visions, disturbing logic, feelings of worthlessness and/or hopelessness and looks that they receive from both loved ones and strangers when they truly believe they are in a type of personal crisis or feel as if they are about to be pushed over the edge. This is just a small portion of what it is like to live with anxiety.

What is Anxiety?

Anxiety, in its simplest form, is a bodily reaction to unfamiliar or dangerous environments and scenarios. Everyone has the tendency to get anxious from time to time and feel distressed or uneasy. This happens perhaps before a big game, performing in front of an audience or right before a huge job interview. Feeling anxious is a natural response that our bodies can feel during moments like these. Anxiety gives us the boost we need to be consciously aware and alert to prepare us for certain situations.

Our body's "fight-or-flight" response is under this umbrella of reactions. But imagine feeling like this *all* the time, even during the calmest of moments?

Picture a life where you have issues concentrating on everyday tasks, where you may be frightened to leave the safety of your home when you cannot fall or stay asleep because your mind is in a constant whirlwind of thought? Living with an anxiety disorder is debilitating. That is putting it lightly in some cases.

Causes of Anxiety

Every one of us is unique, which means even common disorders, like anxiety and depression, resonate within each of us differently, as well as why we are living with anxiety, to begin with. There are several key factors that cause anxiety disorders to grow in the mind:

- Chemistry of the brain
- Environmental factors
- Genetics
- How we grew up
- Life events

The factors listed above are the basics that lay the groundwork to potentially be a victim of anxiety, but those below mixed with any of those above could set one up to be someone that is at a higher risk than others in the development of an anxiety disorder:

- Alcohol, prescription medication or drug abuse
- Chemical imbalances in the body and/or brain
- History of anxiety that runs in family bloodlines
- Occurrence of other mental health issues
- Physical, emotional or mental trauma
- Side effects one has on particular medications
- Stress that lasts an extended amount of time

The feelings and thoughts that anxiety promotes within a sufferer create a bubble that creates lonely thoughts and feelings, which is why it is no surprise that anxiety disorders are the most common of mental illnesses with the U.S, with *over 40 million American adults* living with one of these disorders as we speak.

If it is any consolation, you are by no means alone when it comes to feeling the way you do. There is still a lot of research being put into finding out why anxiety plagues so many individuals, its specific causes and why it resonates within individuals in such vast ways.

Signs & Symptoms of Anxiety Disorders

All of us will experience anxiety in our lives; it is a normal response to stressful life events. But as you have learned so far or experienced for yourself, these symptoms can become much larger than the events of stress them and can interfere heavily with a happy, healthy way of life.

Below are the most common symptoms of anxiety:

- **Worrying** that is disproportionate to the events that trigger it and is intrusive, making it challenging to concentrate on everyday tasks.

- **Agitation** that causes fast heartrates, sweaty hands, dry mouth, etc.

- **Restlessness** or feeling on edge with a constant uncomfortable urge to move that won't go away.

- Becoming **easily fatigued**, either in general or after a panic attack.

- **Difficulty focusing** on everyday tasks.

- **Issues retaining short-term memory** which results in a lack of performance in multiple areas of life.

- Becoming **easily irritable** in the day to day life.

- Constantly having **tense muscles** that may even heighten anxious feelings.

- **Issues falling and staying asleep** due to continued disturbances in the sleep cycle.

- **Panic attacks** that produce overwhelming sensations of fear.

- **Avoidance of social situations** due to a fear of being judged, humiliated, or embarrassed.

- **Extreme fears** about very specific situations or objects that are severe enough to interfere with normal functioning.

Understanding Social Anxiety

Imagine at random times, feeling so uncomfortable in particular situations to the point of not being able to process what is happening around you or difficulty breathing. Welcome to the life of those that deal with social anxiety. Social anxiety is classified by a major discomfort with social interactions as well as a fear of judgment. There are more than 15 million Americans that deal with this in their everyday lives that struggle with the awkwardness of social settings.

Symptoms of Social Anxiety

The main symptoms of this form of anxiety are feeling intensely anxious when in social situations or avoiding them altogether. Many sufferers have a constant feeling that 'something just isn't right', but are never able to pinpoint it.

As you can imagine, these people have a twisted way of thinking that includes false beliefs of situations and negative opinions from others. Many people fear the interaction days or weeks before the event, which means that social anxiety can manifest in other physical symptoms, such as:

- Sweating
- Shaking
- Diarrhea
- Upset stomach
- Muscle tension
- Blushing
- Confusion
- Pounding of heart
- Panic attacks

The key aspect of social anxiety to remember is that even though these folks have a fear of speaking or interacting with others, it doesn't mean they have nothing to say.

Below are things that those who suffer from social anxiety would say to others to help them understand how they feel:

"I do not want this and I cannot help it. It is not just a bit of nervousness that comes and goes. It is constant stress and living in a world that you start to not recognize."

"In my ability to speak right, I lack confidence. There are many times I want to say something, but hold back because I am afraid of how dumb it may sound or that I will be misunderstood. I am afraid of speaking in groups, phone calls, and approaching people the most.

"I am terrified of people's reactions when I do scrounge up the courage to finally speak."

"My anxiety socially is not a constant. There are certain situations that cause me more anxiety than others. It is a fluid disease."

"Many times, people don't realize that those with this anxiety disorder are suffering because of the lack of physical symptoms. Just because you cannot tell there is something wrong, doesn't mean there isn't."

"I cannot help how ridiculous it may seem."

"It hurts to know that people take my anxiety personally instead of just helping me out."

"I wish I had a social life, but my anxiety won't let me; I am not anti-social."

"It may look like I am zoning out from time to time, but I am actually practicing positive self-talk and breathing techniques to stay calm and ward off a panic attack."

"I am not trying to be standoffish, rude, or snobby, even though it may seem that way when I refuse hugs or don't wish to speak. I simply get overwhelmed and overstimulated easily. All I ask for is respect."

"I want people to break the ice and speak to me first. I am genuinely a nice person, I just have a fear I am unable to control."

"I wish more people understood that when I say I cannot come, it is because the situation I was invited to feels 'impossible', not because I don't feel like it."

"When I leave early, I am not being disrespectful. I just need to fight off a meltdown with some alone time."

"Social anxiety is not 'shyness'; that is like comparing a stab wound to a paper cut."
No one experiences social anxiety in the same way. Each day is like living a life of constant fear; worrying about the disapproval of others, rejection, not fitting in, etc. They are bound to be anxious to enter or begin a conversation.

Chapter 2: Acknowledging Your Anxiety

While the numbers of those that suffer from anxiety in the United States alone exceed 40 million, you may feel alone in your symptoms as well as what triggers them. Things that set off those anxious thoughts and feelings are a bit different for everyone who experiences anxiety. It is important to take time to focus on yourself and learn what things provide you with peace or create tension in your life.

Common Anxiety Triggers

- The hustle and bustle of everyday life. Life is always busy and there never seems to be time to slow down.
- The inevitable fact that we are only growing older.
- Driving, especially on freeways with many cars or across bridges.
- Not living up to the expectations that we set for ourselves.
- The sense of uncertainty. When we are not on control of situations we tend to freak out a bit. This comes from a lack of communication and anxiety making conclusions for us.
- Ambulance, fire or police sirens.
- Stresses at work – Not performing well enough, not having enough time during the course of the workday to get things done, etc.
- Simply thinking about what triggers your anxiety can be a cause for anxiousness in itself.
- Being too hot is often times directly associated with being claustrophobic.
- The inevitable part of life known as death. This especially goes for individuals who have experienced much loss in their lives.
- Being alone.

- The possibility of finding out that people do not like you as much as you think they do.
- Being judged or verbally attacked.
- Large crowds.
- The inability to predict the future. Those with anxiety often dislike surprises.
- Trying new things.
- Being far away from home or other places familiar to you.
- When many people speak to or at you all at once.
- The struggles that your children may face at school.
- Money! This is a big one. Whether it is saving for a big event such as a wedding or purchasing a home or car, the process of paying monthly bills while still trying to save money for other things.

Getting to the Root Causes of Your Anxiety

What many of us do not realize is that many causes that trigger our anxieties to flare up are actually self-produced. While you can blame your situation, family, friends, etc. for you distress, you are the one who perceives life as it goes on around you. The way you view it, analyze and take it all is all dependent on you. The root reasons behind the curtains of 'Play Anxiety' are usually caused by one of the following reasons.

Negative Self-Talk

It is said by research conducted by behavioral specialists that upwards of 77% of all the things we think to ourselves is quite counterproductive and negative. What we don't realize is that we are being our own worst critic and a detriment to ourselves. Learn to become consciously aware of the way you speak to yourself.

Write down any sort of negative thoughts for a day and then each day forward practice transforming those negative words or thoughts into a happy, loving one towards yourself. While it may feel weird at first, it will become second nature to you once you practice it for a while. Your self-talk is just as important of a daily habit as any other.

Unrealistic Expectations

Sometimes we simply just have too high of expectations that create a high world that we struggle to reach. Expecting those to be perfect and remember all the details about you is just ridiculous. If your expectations fly way above you, you are more than likely missing out on grand opportunities and are unable to truly recognize the good things that are happening that you should be celebrating.

This goes for the expectations you have for yourself as well. Are they actually realistic? If not, how can you go about making them more reasonable and achievable?

The "Should" Thoughts

Do you find your brain thinking that you "should do this" and you "should do that" often? Have you ever just taken a moment to actually find the reasoning behind why you "should"? Telling yourself that you should is equivalent to telling yourself that you are not good enough. It leads to negative self-talk fast and should be avoided. Make a positive list of the things you should do or become. Are they yours or someone else's expectations?

Taking Things Too Personally

Those with anxiety feel like many things that occur are actually their fault when in reality they more than likely had nothing to do with someone's disgruntled behavior or a glare they received. Learn to not take things too personally because you never know what may be happening in the life of other people.

"We are all in the same game, just different levels. Dealing with the same hell, just at different devils." If you think you are the cause of someone's actions, speak up and ask instead of just assuming. This will get rid of a lot of assumptions that go into negatively feeding your anxiety.

Our minds are wired to believe the things that we tell it the most. If we are always engaging in negative self-talk, expect too much of others or ourselves, do things we just merely think we "should" do or worry about those around you, your brain will act negatively as well. It is all about building a positive foundation for your frame of mind for all those thoughts of yours to dwell in. In order to unlock the door to happiness and less stress and/or anxiety, it is time to get thinking in a happy manner!

Pinpointing Your Anxiety

While you can take all the time in the world to read information in regards to relieving anxiety via the internet, books or other media, unless you take action and decide that you truly want to make a change to lower your anxiousness, it will never happen. I am an anxiety sufferer and back just a couple years ago it engulfed my everyday life and drowned me more than a few times.

I finally over time came up with a process that assisted me greatly with determining what triggered my anxious thoughts so that I could get a grip on my life and yield them from continuously taking over my personal life.

- *Stop* – When those feeling of anxiousness begin to hit you, stop and take a moment to make a mental note of what you are doing right at that moment. This is easier said than done, for you might be in the middle of a task, conversation, etc. But it is beneficial to take just a moment to identify when you began to feel anxious.

- *Identify* – Recognizing the onset of anxiety will help you come to the conclusion of what actually causes it for you personally. If you develop the capability to notice triggers and feelings when they start to dwell, you can put a stop to them faster. Many people don't realize they are feeling anxious until their symptoms are outrageously taking over them. Over time, you will be able to catch on more quickly what is threatening your happiness and overall well-being.

- **Write** – As you become an expert of taking moments to make mental notes of why you feel anxious, I find that at the end of the day I write down the events during my day, both the goods one and those that triggered my anxiety. I keep a notepad on my cellular device so that I am quickly able to access it to jot down notes at the moment and then write them down on paper before heading to bed. Be sure to write down as many details as possible – what you are thinking, experiencing and feeling, etc.

- **Analyze** – At the end of the week is when I choose to review what I have written in my anxiety notebook. You can review it at the end of each day, week or month, but I do not recommend waiting any longer than that. I wait at least a couple days to a week so that I can see the pattern that my thoughts made. When you are aware of these patterns you are better able to focus on the causes of anxiety and avoid them.

- **Possibilities** – There are numerous things that you can make the scapegoat when it comes to feeling anxious. If you have adequate knowledge of these ideas, you can review patterns and conquer anxiety. Anxiety in many cases is situational. If you are anxious being in unfamiliar surroundings, expose yourself to these types of circumstances a little time. If your causes are more based on the way you think and view the world, learn to engage in positive self-talk. Once you have a pattern written out, you will be less anxious just by the fact that you have some idea and control over your anxiety situation overall.

Chapter 3: Trauma and Anxiety

The journey of life is exciting, scary, ridiculous, confusing and worth it all at once. But there are times that we all go through some type of emotional distress, whether it be mere sadness, rapid anxiety, addictions to outside influences, obsessions with things or people, compulsions we have a hard time controlling, behaviors that are self-sabotaging, physical injuries, anger, and bleak moods, among the hundreds of other things we go through, think and/or feel.

It is important to learn ways to cope when it comes to hard times, no matter the time frame. Something psychologically downgrading can happen in a matter of mere moments and leave you scarred for the rest of your life. Some people seek out help from other individuals who are professionals at understanding the human mind, but others wish to find help within them. Having the knowledge to help yourself is not an easy feat. It may be easy to read pages upon pages of books and self-help websites that provide information, but it is much harder to put those words into actions.

The world is a much different place now than it was just a decade or two ago. Technology has advanced so rapidly that some of us are overwhelmed with it all, especially the consequences that we receive, whether from our own actions or that of another being who acted upon a current mood. Human beings are not the robots that we seem to want to create so badly these days. We are emotionally driven individuals with a lack of having the knack to help ourselves in times of need and/or trouble.

The worst thing about the constant rise of this distress is the fact that there is no one age group or certain targeted individuals that are more likely to go through it. It is happening clear from late grade school levels all the ways into senior living years. Students have much more stress with perpetual levels of testing and pressure to be better. Employees live their hard-earned careers always fighting to make their way up the ladder with not much reward. Older individuals are continuously having their wages and retirement that they worked their entire lives for whisked away.

It is a dog eat dog world out there with a lot of room to make mistakes that can cause even more friction in our personal lives. With the constant pressure to be better than the next, our society has taught us maybe how to be more proficient in terms of getting things done at school or work, but many of us have forgotten the person that is truly important: OURSELVES. If we do not take care of our emotional health, detrimental things can occur. Below are some signs that you may be experiencing emotional distress. Some of the symptoms may surprise you.

Childhood Trauma and Sensitivity to Anxiety

Trauma during childhood can impact our entire lives. According to the Journal of Affective Disorders, children who experience traumatic situations are much more likely to have anxiety and depressions and fall victim to alcohol and drug abuse. The same study found that females are more susceptible than males to develop anxiety, even with the same rates of trauma.

If left untreated, trauma during childhood can have effects that last throughout someone's entire life. They are likely to developmental disorders that branch out to much more than just anxiety as well.

Common Anxiety Disorders Caused by Trauma

Common anxiety disorders that are caused by traumatic events are:

- Panic disorder
- Obsessive Compulsive Disorder (OCD)
- Post-Traumatic Stress Disorder (PTSD)
- Body Dysmorphic Disorder

- Agoraphobia
- Social Phobia(s)

As you can imagine, trauma anytime throughout your life can play a major part in the development of anxiety and other mental disorders in your lifetime.

Chapter 4: Grabbing your life back from anxiety

Now that you have acknowledged that life could be better and have learned how to interpret why you live a life filled with anxiety, it is time to take your life back, pronto! There is a variety of methods we will discuss in this chapter that can help you gain back the confidence you need to live life to the fullest.

Managing Your Emotions

Emotions are a natural human phenomenon. , and are very present in pressing and painful times. Every day we are driven by some force of emotions:

- We take chances because we get excited about new opportunities
- We cry because we are hurting and make sacrifices for those we love

Those are just a couple examples of emotions; they dictate our actions, intentions, and thoughts with authority to our rational minds. Emotions can become a real problem, however, when we act too fast or we act on wrong types of emotions, which cause us to make rash decisions.

Negative emotions, such as bitterness, envy, or rage, are the ones that tend to spiral out of control the most, especially when triggered. It only takes one slip of our emotions to totally screw up the relationships in our lives.

If you have issues controlling your emotions, here are some steps that you can implement into your everyday life that will help you regain rationality, no matter what challenging situation you are facing:

Don't react right away

You are more likely to make mistakes when you react right away to emotional triggers. When reacting right away to these triggers, you are likely to say and do things that you will later regret.

Before acting on emotions, take a deep breath to stabilize your impulses.

Breathe deeply for just a couple minutes and you will be able to feel your heart rate return to normal. One you become calmer, remind yourself that feeling this way is just temporary.

Find healthy outlets

Once you have managed your emotions, you need to learn how to release that build up in the healthiest way possible; emotions are something that you should never let bottle up. Talk to someone you trust. Hearing their opinion of the matter can help to broaden your thoughts and regain control.

Many people keep a journal to write down how they feel. Others engage in exercise to discharge their emotions. Others meditate in order to return to their tranquil state. Whatever activity suits you, find it and use it when emotions get high.

Look at the bigger picture

All happenings in our, both bad and good, serves a purpose in our lives. Being able to see past the moment strengthens your wisdom. You may not understand certain circumstances right away, but over time, you will see the bigger picture as the pieces of the puzzle fall into order. Even when in an emotionally upsetting time, trust that there is a reason that you will comprehend in time.

Replace your thoughts

Negatively fueled emotions create negative recurring thoughts that create cycles of negative patterns over time. When confronted with these emotions, force them out of your mind and replace them with more positive thoughts. Visualize the ideal ending playing out or think about someone or something that makes you happy.

Forgive your triggers

Triggers could be the ones you love the most; you're best friend(s), your family, yourself, etc. There will be times that you may feel a sudden wave of rage when people do things that annoy you or a self-loathing feeling when you remember back to the past when you could have done thing differently. The key to managing your emotions is to first, forgive. This allows you to detach from your jealousy, fury, and resentment. As you forgive, you will discover that disassociating yourself from these feelings will do you the best.

Every day we are constantly reminded of how strong and prominent our emotions are and the power they have. We are bound to take the wrong action from time to time and feel the wrong things. To avoid acting out, simply take a few steps back and calm your spirit that is heightened from outside forces. You will be grateful for mastering your emotions when it comes to building and strengthening meaningful relationships.

Using the Power of Mini Habits

Just after Christmas in the days ending 2016, I was reflecting on the year. I realized that I had tons of room to improve but always failed at keeping up with my New Year's resolutions. Instead, I decided that in 2017, I would explore other options.

On the 28th of December, I made the choice that I wanted to get back in shape. Previously, I hardly if ever exercised and had a consistent guilt about it. My goal was a 30-minute workout, realistic, right?

I found myself unmotivated, tired, and the guilt made me feel worthless. It wasn't until a few days later that I came across a small blog article about thinking the opposite of the ideas you are stuck on. The clear opposite of my 30-minute workout goal was chilling on the couch, stuffing my face with junk food, but my brain went to the idea of 'size.'

What if, instead of carrying that guilty feeling around all the time, I just performed one push-up? I know, right? How absurd of me to think that a single push-up would do anything to help me towards my goal.

What I found was a magical secret to unlocking my potential…when I found myself struggling with my bigger goals; I gave in and did a push-up. Since I was already down on the floor, I did a few more. Once I performed a few, my muscles felt warmed up and I decided to attempt a pull-up. As you can imagine, I did several more. And soon, I exercised for entire 30-minutes!

What Are Mini Habits?

Mini habits are just like they sound; you choose a habit you want to change and you shrink them down to stupidly small tasks.

For instance, if you want to start writing at least 1,000 words per day:

- Write 50 words per day

- Read two pages of a book per day

Easy, right? I could accomplish this in 10 to 20 minutes or so. You will find that once you start meeting this daily requirement, you will far exceed them faster than you would imagine.

What is *More* Essential than Your *Habits*?

You might be wondering how you can become more comfortable in your skin and be yourself in a cruel world with these so-called mini habits. Well, think about it; what is more important than the things you do each and every day? NOTHING. Habits are responsible for 45% of how we behave, making up the foundation of who we are and how happy we are in life.

The main reason people fail to change anything in their life, even the aspects they know need to change is because they never instill new habits. Why? Simply because in the past, they have tried to do way too much, all at once. If establishing a new habit requires you to have more willpower than you can muster, you are bound to be unsuccessful. If a habit requires less willpower, you are much more likely to succeed!

Benefits of Mini Habits

There are many additional benefits that come with utilizing mini habits in your everyday life. Here are a few:

- Consistent success breeds more success
- No more guilt
- Stronger productivity
- Formation of more positively impactful habits
- Generation of motivation

Chapter 5: Belittle anxiety with personal empowerment

Having a negative attitude towards life keeps us from being happy and impacts those that we interact daily with. Science has more than enough proof to show how being positive impacts your levels of happiness and terms of success. This is why making positivity a habit with the help of small changes can help you to drastically change your overall life and the mindset you have towards the world. The life you are living is a direct reflection of your overall attitude. It can be quite easy, almost too easy, to be cynical at the world and see it as a mess of injustice and tragedy, especially thanks to the media that we all spend many hours a day on.

Negativity is holding you back from really enjoying your life and has a great impact on your environment as well. The energy that people bring to the table, including you, is very contagious. One of the best things you can do in your life that is free of charge and simplistic is to offer your positive attitude. This is especially beneficial in a world that loves and craves negativity.

One of my favorite quotes of all time comes directly from the King of Pop, Michael Jackson: *"If you want to make the world a better place, take a look at yourself and make a change."*

As humans, we are creatures of habit. In this chapter, we will outline small but significant changes that can be made to form positive habits that can drastically change the overall mindset of your life around.

Smile

When asked who we think about most of the time, the most honest answer would probably have to be ourselves, right? This is natural, so don't feel guilty! It is good to hold ourselves accountable and take responsibility for ourselves.

But I want to challenge you to put yourself aside for at least one moment per day (I recommend striving for more) and make another person smile.

Think about making someone else happy and that warm feeling you get when you receive happiness. We don't realize how intense the impact of making someone smile can have on those around us. Plus, smiling costs nothing and positively works your facial muscles!

Focus on solutions, not problems

Embracing positivity doesn't mean you need to avoid issues, but rather it is learning how to reconstruct the way you criticize. Those that are positive create criticisms with the idea to improve something. If you are just going to point out the issues with people and in situations, then you should learn to place that effort instead into suggesting possible solutions. You will find that pointing out solutions makes everyone feel more positive than pointing out flaws.

Notice the rise, not just the downfall

Many of us are negative just by the simple fact that we dwell too much on the hate and violence that is in our daily media. But what we fail to notice is those that are rising up, showing compassion, and giving love to others. Those are the stories you should engulf yourself in. When you able to find modern-day heroes in everyday life, you naturally feel more hopeful, even in tough times.

Just breathe

Our emotions are connected to the way we breathe. Think about a time that you held your breath when you were in deep concentration or when you are upset or anxious. Our breath is dependent on how we feel, which means it also has the power to change our emotions too!

Fend off other's negativity

I'm sure you have gone to work cheerful and excited to take on the day ahead, but then your co-worker ruins that happy-go-lucky mood of yours with their complaints about every little thing, from the weather to other employees, to their weekend, etc.

It is natural to find yourself agreeing to what others are saying, especially if you like to avoid conflict. But you are initially allowing yourself to drown in their pool of negative emotions. Don't fall into this trap.

Conflict may arise, but I challenge you to not validate the complaints of a friend, family member, or co-worker next time they are going about on a complaint-spree. They are less likely to be negative in the future if they have fewer people to complain to.

Switch the "*I have to*" mindset with "*I get to*"

I am sure you often fail to notice how many times we tell ourselves that we have to go and do something.

- "I have to go to work."
- "I have to go to the store."
- "I have to pay rent."
- "I have to mow the lawn."

You get the picture. But watch what happens when you swap the word have with the word get.

- "I get to go to work."
- "I get to go to the store."
- "I get to pay rent."
- "I get to mow the lawn."

See the change in attitude there? It goes from needing to fulfill those obligations to be grateful that you have those things to do in your life. This means:

- You have a job to go to
- You have enough money to support yourself and your family to provide a healthy meal
- You have a roof over your head
- You have a nice yard

When you make this simple change, you will begin to feel the warmth of happiness snuggle you like the cold blanket of stress falls away.

Describe your life positively

The choice of vocabulary we use has much more power over our lives than we realize. How you discuss your life is essential to harnessing positivity since your mind hears what you spew out loud.

When you describe your life as boring, busy, chaotic, and/or mundane, this is exactly how you will continue to perceive it and it will directly affect both your mental and physical health.

Instead, if you describe your life as involved, lively, familiar, simple, etc., you will begin to see changes in your overall perspective and you will find more joy in the way you choose to mold your entire life.

Master rejection

You will need to learn to become good at being rejected. The fact of the matter is, rejection is a skill. Instead of viewing failed interviews and broken hearts as failures, see them as opportunities for practice to ensure you are ready for what is to come next. Even if you try to avoid it, rejection is inevitable. Don't allow it to harden you from the inside out.

Rethink challenges

Stop picturing your life being scattered with dead-end signs and view all your failings as opportunities to re-direct. There are little to no things in life that we have 100-percent control over. When you let uncontrollable experiences take over your life, you will literally turn into mush.

What you can control is the amount of effort you put into things without an ounce of regret doing them! When you are able to have fun taking on challenges, you are embracing adventure and the unknown, which allows you much more room to grow, learn and win in the future.

Write in a gratitude journal

There are bound to be days where just one situation can derail the entire day, whether it be an interaction that is not so pleasant or something that happens the night before the day ahead, our mind clings to these negative aspects of the day.

I am sure you have read on multiple sites about how keeping a gratitude journal is beneficial. If you are anything like me, I thought this was total rubbish that is until I started doing it. I challenged myself to write down at least five things that I was truly grateful for each and every day. Scientifically, expressing gratitude is linked to happiness and reducing stress.

I challenge you to begin jotting down things you appreciate and are grateful for each day. Even on terrible days, there is something to be blessed about!

Chapter 6: Everyday techniques to fend off anxiety

Despite the toll that anxiety and its symptoms can have on everyday life and fulfillment, in today's world there are many different techniques and methods you can learn to incorporate into your everyday routine that help you to control and possibly even eliminate anxiety from your life. Each section of this chapter will be dedicated to a specific genre of techniques that anyone has the ability to learn!

Visualization and Anxiety

Seeing *is* believing, which is a key secret to how entrepreneurs and well-known people in society stand out and achieve success and fulfill their dreams. ***Visualization is the simple use of imagination through mental imagery to help form visions of what we want in our lives and how we can make them a reality.***

There are two main kinds of visualization:

Pragmatic Visualization represents a set of days that helps to gain new ideas and interpret what it says/means to them. It helps those understand structures that lie within a set of data.

Artistic Visualization is similar to pragmatic in that it utilizes visuals to convey information but in a different sense. It is used to show people that data is being monitored carefully and shows particular aspects of data that is connected to one another to depict an entire idea.

So, how does learning about these two kinds of visualization help you in your quest to decrease anxiety? Well, visual techniques help to drastically overcome symptoms of anxiety. When the two types are combined, visualization is powerful in obtaining and staying in a calmer state of mind.

When it comes to anxiety, visualization requires one to picture themselves in a safe, peaceful and/or tranquil environment. Anywhere that makes you happier is where you should be imagining yourself during visualization exercises. It does sound pretty funny at first glance, but trust me when I say there is something about being able to transport your mind to somewhere mentally tranquil. Not only will your mind thank you but your body will too, for it becomes much more relaxed and stress-free when performing these practices. Visualization gives people something to distract themselves from the current world that surrounds them.

Why You Should Be Using Visualization

Beyond visualization itself, you can literally view the best of life from the comfort of your own couch. This chapter will showcase the benefits that come with the dedicated practice of learning and incorporating ways of visualization into your everyday life.

- **Improved quality of relationships** – The positive outcomes of utilizing visualization doesn't just end within yourself. Since you are developing a better mindset that aids in your views and beliefs, those around you will like and appreciate the more confident, positive you!

- **Boosts your mood** – When one practices the methods of visualization, they naturally experience a sort of joy that is quite unexplainable to some. Once you finish one of these sessions successfully, you will more than likely feel boastfully happy, calm and relaxed.

- **Relieves stress** – Practicing the ways of visualization naturally causes one to be able to relax. It has a way of quieting the mind to be able to think happier, more positive thoughts which tone down loads of stress that pile on our shoulders almost on a daily basis.

- **Strengthens the immune system** – Thanks to all that dialing down

168

of stress and things that fuel stress, your body is better able to fight off sickness which makes you physically better, longer. This also helps in aiding anxiety because you are not constantly worrying about getting ill all the time as well.

- **Ability to learn new things quicker** – When the mind is in a calmer state, it is able to pick up and grasp new concepts much easier than when it is bogged down with so many negative thoughts and emotions.

- **Able to cope with the feeling of nervousness** – When you take time out of your day to practice visualization, you are initially settling all those negative feelings that you may have about yourself and what others may think of you as well. This immensely helps individuals who are naturally more nervous combat that feeling, which leaves room to try and experiment with new things and ideas. Imagine yourself in a great looking outfit giving that inevitable speech that is due soon. Then imagine an applauding audience. It is quite the confidence booster!

- **Builds stronger concentration skills** – Visualization makes room for your mind to do other tasks efficiently by spring cleaning negative thoughts, feelings, emotions, and past experiences. This doesn't mean it is responsible for getting rid of them 100%, but it helps one to be able to cope and bring down those bad levels to make room for productivity.

- **Assists in overcoming recurring issues** – When the weight of your entire world is upon your shoulders, it is no wonder that we begin to believe that our lives were just made to be a laughing-stalk to some because of how life's unlucky events have left us feeling. This can lead to long-term problems and beliefs. Visualization combats these two things.

- **Can give you a spark of inspiration** – During your sessions, if your mind always veers to one idea in particular, perhaps it is time to take initiative and proceed with the steps in achieving it! Visualizing doing something can directly inspire you to do as such.

- **Makes one more creative** – Visualization not only takes concentration but also a truckload of creativity as well. If you are going to picture something in detail and add the other four senses to that visual, you have to really want to mold it into reality. We all have creative bones in our bodies. Visualization just brings them out more, honing that skill and letting it shine.

- **No boundaries** – As I have mentioned before, when it comes to visualization, practice makes perfect. Just like with any newly acquired skill, one must learn to hone its practice to be able to tweak it when needed and use it to their utmost advantage. With certain visualization techniques, you can literally picture yourself doing something that would otherwise be usually hard to achieve. With those images in mind, you then have a good idea what you must do to actually and realistically accomplish that image you had in your head during a visualization session. This method knows no bounds!

- **Method of practice and rehearsal** – Believe it or not, visualization can be a way to practice your favorite sport or nail that upcoming work pitch that you have been reciting and memorizing for days. Picturing yourself doing or performing something is just as effective as actually completing the task at hand. Utilizing visualization with real, physical practice can get you to honing that skill or memorizing things much quicker.

- **Picture yourself getting stronger and healthier** – Sounds unbelievable, but if you are sick, seeing yourself get better will have the result of getting healthier, sooner. Visualization reduces stress and relaxes your mind, which also assists in healing your body of sickness or physical injury as well. This allows your body to function at its full capacity. You would be surprised what our bodies could accomplish in a day's work if we treated them more like the temples they are and should always be. It is safe to say we take our physical presence for granted most days. And it tends to show more often than not!

- **Gives us joy** – Many people who practice the ways of visualization tend to picture something that brings them happiness. We almost are never quite in the right place or time in our lives to always have what we want and that is okay! But that doesn't mean we shouldn't get the luxury of seeing it for ourselves, right? Picturing a goal or what we want the most from life can bring us quite a load of temporary happiness if one wants to view it that way. Why temporary? If you can picture it, you can eventually and more than likely make it happen in your future, which is why visualization can be a great motivator.

Aspects of Successful Visualization Practices

There are three aspects to successfully become one with visualization:

- **Practice** – Learning the ways of visualization may actually be more stressful and frustrating for beginners because it is not a practice we are naturally keen to perform. Those that start practicing visualization have a false sense of what the experience is supposed to feel like and have false expectations about the outcome. This inhibits the practice from really taking effect. Visualization is something that has to be practiced daily to work for you long-term. If practiced the right way, it will eventually become second nature to you but only if you really dedicate yourself to learning its ways and practicing it every day until you have it down pat.

- **Utilizes ALL the senses** – Visualization doesn't just use your sense of how a certain peaceful place appears to you in your mind. You have to imagine what your safe space smells, tastes sounds and feels like as well. The more detailed you are in regards to your senses, the better visualization you will have and the more relaxed you can potentially become.

- **Actions** – All human beings experience mental barriers that keep them from being happy and the process of practicing and performing visualization is not excluded from this. Even for visualizing experts, bad thoughts from the course of one's day can inhibit one from getting a clear vision of their safe haven. You have to find a way to release and/or transform those bad thoughts and feelings into something that you can tangibly get rid of.

Forms of Visualization for Anxiety

Visualization is a skill that can be utilized to obtain a better life, especially for those that suffer from an anxiety disorder. Now, we will talk about techniques in the visualization world. Although all of these are not for everyone, try them out and see what works for you.

Meditation

Meditation is a superb form of apathetic visualization that can lead to very powerful results. Visualizing through means of meditation is more of an outgrowth than the main focus. When you begin to incorporate meditation sessions into your everyday routine, you will gradually be opening the door to your inner self, which will then lead you to be able to visualize more clearly and easily.

The more experience you have with meditation, the smoother sessions become and the more you get to see and take away from your visions. It is important not to become frustrated with yourself or discouraged from continuing to practice meditation if you are just starting out.

The whole point of meditation is to empty your brain of thoughts and feelings and to let your mind wander to wherever it wants to go. A vital component of meditation is breathing. Learn to focus on how you take in and let out breaths of air. Let your mind veer off to wherever its little heart desires. Once you begin to practice this technique more often, it will become easier and faster to exhaust your mind of concerns or other worries and let other things come in and explore. It will become second nature for you to sit down, relax and get into a clear state of mind so that you can visualize to your contentment.

Meditation makes way for things that you never thought were actually within you. Once you rid your brainwaves of all that noise from the course of your day, thoughts occur at their own pace.

Altered Memory Visualization

This visualization technique targets past memories and learning how to change them to a more positive standpoint. For those with anxiety about things that stem from their past, this is especially helpful in obtaining a brighter state of mind. This technique is one to utilize if you are one that holds on to past anger and resentment from particular situations that you finally want to rid yourself of.

No one can change the past, but you can teach your brain how it views these past scenarios in your mind. Get into a calmed state and visualize the scenario that you wish had a different outcome. Restore things said that were fueled by anger with comments that are controlled and peaceful. This does take some time and you may have to revisit this scene in your head multiple times to nail the outcome that you wish had resulted from the past situation. It is recommended to not do this day upon day in a row, but rather space out revisiting the scene.

Over time, your brain will begin to only recall what YOU have recreated, making a once painful or uncomfortable situation fade away in memory. Try to imagine little cubicle offices in each major section of your brain. In this instance, I like to picture a little office guy that is in charge of just the bad memories. During these sessions, you are instructing him on how to rewrite particular events that have occurred in the past and once they are rewritten the way you once anticipated them to play out, this office dude can start to shred your memories of these occurrences.

Receptive Visualization

This technique is much like viewing a movie inside your head, but you are the director of the scenes within this movie. Get yourself to a quiet space, lie back, get comfortable and close your eyes. Focus on building the scene in which you want to see acted out in your mind.

Once a clear backdrop and scenery is within your mind, place people, noises, smells and sounds within your scene of this movie. It is best to slowly build your way up to the actual scene until you are comfortable and content with it, then it is time for action! Focus on feeling involved within this scene of your "movie."

Treasure Map

This visualization technique not only uses mental fundamentals but also physical components as well. You will need to have an idea of what you want to visualize before getting to the nitty-gritty of performing this method. Start by using your art skills to draw out some type of physical representation of the components you need to achieve in order to reach your ultimate goal.

For example, perhaps you have an upcoming test that you want to get a great grade on. Draw out a building symbolizes a school, a book that you will need to use to study for this test and then a representation of yourself. Try to make your drawing detailed, but do not worry about the maturity of your art abilities too much here. It is not the drawings themselves that are important, but rather what you are imagining WHILE sketching them out.

As you draw out your "map to success", your mind is actually visualizing ways that will get you to where you want to be. Patience is a key with this particular technique, for it does take a bit of time to truly become completely mentally occupied in this exercise. It is crucial to take your notepad and pen to a quiet space and to not be around anything distracting such as a radio, television, people or phones.

How to Design Your Own "Safe Space"

Safe places or spaces are a mind's sanctuary, created for the purpose of retreat if one needs a mental location to be able to visualize or hone their meditative state and reduce stress. Creating one of these is kind of like personalizing a physical space in your home. You want to do anything to truly make it YOURS.

It can be anything from a room inside an imaginary home, a room in your realistic home that you want to visualize differently, the beach, a comforting outdoorsy area, etc. As you meditate or relax and begin to dive deeper into your imagery or visualization session, this is the place you imagine you want to go. It is anywhere that you wish to return to time after time, so put some effort and thought into where you will always find comfort in mentally retreating to.

- **Brainstorm** – The goal is to develop a place that you feel calm, content and happy within, no matter the reason that you retreat to it. If you have difficulty seeking out such a place, start by looking through art, magazines, books, old photographs, etc. Always lean towards ideas that burst with positivity for you.

- Are you more apt to feel calmer in an outdoor/natural setting or do you feel better within the walls of some type of structure?

- Are there pieces of writing such as within books, poems of stories that make you feel at ease?

- Do you feel more comforted by populated areas or tranquil areas?

- **Think of a time where you felt happy and safe** – Memories are the best areas to seek things that bring joy to you. Think back to memories that you were happy, content, playful, peaceful, etc. Write these down in detail. It could be literally anywhere, as long as it brought contentment to you.

  - Where did this memory occur?
  - How old were you?
  - Why did this memory make you happy?
  - Who was with you within this memory?

- **Create various rooms** – Your safe space does not necessarily have to be just 2D, one room vision. It can have various sections, compartments or rooms within it. This allows you to trek to different areas throughout your visualization sessions. This also allows one the ability to be able to compartmentalize issues and deal with them one part at a time.

  - *Fill your space with cherished people* – There are many individuals that would rather be alone while in their safe place, while others prefer the company of their favorite people. Imagine who makes you happy and during the course of a visualization session, imagine greeting them and welcoming them into your safe space. This also goes for people in your life that may have passed away that you miss and wish to see. Having conversations with them and asking for advice could make a world of difference!

- *Utilize ALL your senses* – Seeing is believing, but visions of your safe place are a lot more believable and turn in better results if you learn to engage all your senses while within them. Engulf yourself in tastes, sounds smells and how things feel between your fingers and toes and against your skin. It will enhance your visualization experience ten-fold.

- *Write out all the details* – Once you have taken the dedicated time to develop and build your safe place, write down all the tiniest details that you can remember. Writing in a lot of detail can assist you in returning to that place in your mind easier and more efficiently. Some individuals even videotape, sculpt, draw or paint out their descriptions for safekeeping for future use.

  - Are there animals or people?
  - What do you feel?
  - How small or big is your space?
  - What colors?
  - What surrounds you?
  - What is the ultimate backdrop or setting?

- **Visualize positive results** – The main rule of thumb for visualization is imagining situations acted out in positive manners. This involves a heavy amount of thinking happily and setting up a content scene. Imaging positive outcomes are really just a more in-depth version of regular run-of-the-mill positive thinking.

Developing Anxiety Routines

Anxiety routines are any type of daily routine that you use to calm yourself down in stressful situations and that leaves you feeling physical, mental or emotionally distressed. These routines are meant to help you bounce back from the depths of your own thoughts and live a life full of more passion and fulfillment.

This means it is very crucial to choose routines that not only suit you but are healthy, too. Life runs smoother when you have a routine to fulfill those nasty little voices in your head or when you feel like you may make a bad choice because of your anxiety symptoms. Sadly, some people choose unhealthy habitual routines that not only push them back into a negative state but may even provoke symptoms of anxiety and make them worse.

These bad routines could be anything from drug use, both illegal and prescription, large consumption of alcohol or heavy smoking of cigarettes, etc. You get the picture. Creating an anxiety routine for yourself should not include things that will cause you greater harm in the long run. Honestly, habits like those stated above are only going to make your symptoms worse.

As human beings, we are automatically wired to detect any sort of negative energy that may cause us harm. Anxiety becomes so bad within certain people simply because our bodies do not quite know the difference between stressful triggers that are actually harmless to us versus actual, life-threatening aspects that may be sprung upon us.

Our bodies are made to react to protect ourselves. This is why being mentally prepared for the day that lies ahead of you is so crucial, especially for anxiety sufferers. It is important to back up our thoughts with an extra layer of positivity to promote a sense of safety and well-being. This is much easier said than done, especially when life may not have been a very good friend to you as of late. But being able to mentally develop a positive sense of self is the first step in creating daily routines that help pave your way to a successful life to live and your future.

Routines to Decrease Anxiety

With the right amount of inspiration, the first day or two of adding a new routine to your life can be exciting. You know you are making a positive change that will hopefully help you feel better about yourself and the life you live. However, self-care routines can be a hard thing to manage and utilize on a regular basis once the newness of acting upon it wears off.

Anxiety can leave some sufferers so dismayed by anxious or sad thoughts that they want nothing more than to do away with anything that resonates positive energy. But this is the exact opposite of fighting for yourself and your happiness. Everyone has their bad days and moments and by all means, you are allowed to have and live those. But it is important not to stay tucked away in them for long periods of time.

Developing and executing specific daily routines that you are comfortable with gives those a step by step plan for the day and keeps you prepared for situations or other anxiety triggers from leaping out and mugging you of your happiness. Routines, kind of like exercise, are things we practice daily to keep us in shape, but anxious routines keep our minds in check. You never know when something will catch you off guard, when a person may ask you something that is bothersome or when a debilitating symptom of anxiety will hit you throughout the course of the day. It is better to be prepared than not to be, right?

The Importance of a Balanced Morning Routine

Many functions within routines do them absolutely no good. When the alarm goes off, they tend to hit snooze a few times. When they finally decide to open their eyes, they automatically reach for their phones and look at updates on social media. Many people are already let down by the fact no one messaged them or liked their posts throughout the night.

When their feet finally touch the floor to stand up out of bed, they are already on a path to a negative, self-destructing day. They take a quick shower, down a bowl of cereal and chug a cup of coffee and get to their day job...what is the point?

This lack of routine is non-beneficial. We see our unstructured lives as having no real purpose, which results in a lack of inner peace. We are destroying our happiness without realizing it!

Benefits of a Morning Routine

Creating a morning routine is not only a big part in relieving anxiety, but it also boosts productivity, brings out your inner positivity, helps you to develop and successfully sustain good relationships, as well as being a big reducer of negativities. Morning routines alone have been shown to be the best strategy for reducing stress and relieving those pesky symptoms of anxiety, no matter how long they have resided within you.

Morning routines keep you consciously aware and more grounded throughout the day. In fact, many who were once stubborn and did not want to incorporate a daily routine were eventually surprised at how much better they felt each and every morning. Anxiety levels dropped and confidence and happiness levels substantially rose. A morning routine can literally reduce your anxiety by as much as sixty percent!

Steps to Include in Your Morning Routine

When you **wake up earlier,** you know that you have plenty of time to get up and get ready for your day, which aids in decreased stress levels. If there is adrenaline pumping throughout your body as you rush around to head out the door, it sticks with you for the rest of the day.

Sounds like a waste of time, but **making your bed each morning** is a powerful task that helps you gain the momentum you need to get pumped for the day ahead. For those that suffer from anxiety and depression, making the bed is simple but can make a huge difference because you know you have completed *one* task if not anything else.

Meditation and prayer is a subject with many critics. People view meditation as an act performed only by spiritual individuals. Practicing mindfulness daily has positive side effects that can trigger feel-good hormones in the brains that aid in reducing levels of stress, anxiety and even depression.

Mixing meditation and prayer within your morning routine can be quite vitalizing, giving clarity to your life and your decisions. If you wish to learn more about the power behind the act of prayer, it will be covered in the following chapter The Empowerment of Prayer.

Taking an ice cold shower in the mornings has been proven to provide the human body with a great number of benefits. Cold exposure, also known as cold shower therapy, is nothing new. Our ancestors utilized it as a remedy to treat mental ailments. Showering in cold water provides the body with adequate circulation and tones the skin nicely.

The cold feeling kicks positive responses throughout the body into overdrive. It accelerates the repairing of cells, which reduces inflammation, pain, and speeds up our metabolic processes. The icy waters help lower negative levels that depression and anxiety can hover over us. Standing under the cold water for just a couple minutes can yield you these benefits.

Substitute your breakfast with coffee or tea to bump up energy levels and replace your usual breakfast eats. This is not recommended for absolutely everyone, but if you are trying to find ways to keep hunger away for the first portion of your day, give it a shot!

Learn how to **utilize a journal** to make "morning pages" as part of your routine in the mornings. This is my personal favorite way to "mind dump" any curious or troubling thoughts you had during the previous day and the night before, as well as random ideas that pop into your mind. I write in my journal after taking a shower, since great ideas tend to spring during those few minutes. When you are able to write down all the negative feelings on paper, you can then get through the day with a clearer state of mind.

Practice gratitude by jotting down things you would miss if they were no longer in your life, such as objects, people, etc. into your morning pages.

To start the day on a positive note, **jot down what you are looking forward** to that day. This tells our brains to look up, think up and be bright and helps to relieve anxiety.

Write down your intentions at the beginning of each day, no matter how corny they may sound, such as *"I will choose to be consciously present today."*

Write out important tasks that you wish to achieve during the day to ensure you will feel prepared and have a fulfilling plan. This will ease your mind so that you can develop a clear path of action to achieving that days' goals.

I know I have mentioned writing a lot, but like I said before it is a powerful tool. Every morning our brains are ready to go and on high alert, so it is good to have a well-thought-out plan of action.

Write down at least three to five of the most important tasks that you have to complete. Focus on ones that stress you out just thinking about them. Then, ask yourself the following questions about the tasks you have jotted out so that you can prioritize them accordingly:

- Which tasks will help me inch closer to achieving my main goal?

- What task do I have the most fearful anxious thoughts about?

- Which tasks have the potential to cancel out others if done successfully?

Spend 90 minutes every day working towards accomplishing your priorities. Targeting your main goals during the morning hours help you to get them accomplished productively.

Other Morning Methods to Relieve Anxiety

Play uplifting music to ensure an upbeat, positive mood. Create a playlist to play throughout your morning routine. Make your phone's alarm tone a good song to wake up to. You would be surprised at what a difference this effortless step takes.

Spend time with a pet(s) to help raise your dopamine and serotonin levels, resulting in lessened anxiety and depression. Pets also motivate us to climb out of bed and give us the initiative to take on the day, even when our anxiety tries to get the best of us. Adding them to your morning routine is a bonus for not only you but for your pet's well-being too!

Change your scenery in simple ways; Go outside, take a walk. Visit your favorite café and grab a coffee. Go out with a friend. The longer you dwell in a space that sucks away happiness, the worse you will feel.

Interactions with the outside world can be enough to distract you from your anxious habits. This is another reason routines are so important in aiding anxiety. Avoiding responsibilities can actually damage you mentally more than you realize. It is good to get your attention off the darkness of life that resides inside your head. It only makes your anxiety worse when you sit around and obsess over it.

Coping with anxiety and its symptoms can lead to a life of great discomfort. Having some type of structure in the form of routines can be quite crucial to one's success in living a happy, go-lucky life. The next few chapters will cover other types of routines in detail that can help relieve and maybe even make your symptoms disappear for good! It is all about you to initiate making the change.

Chapter 7: Transforming Your anxiety for a better life

If you are feeling anxious or depressed about your future and are allowing negative thoughts to get the best of you and dampen your motivation for success, then learning to use anxiety to your advantage is a must.

Personally, I have learned to *choose* to view my anxiety has a valuable asset that yields me to lead a more authentic life. I live empathetically, for my anxiety has made me a vulnerable person and thus, helped me deepen my life's relationships.

Having anxiety just means I am not mellow enough to take things for granted in life, therefore, making life a richer experience all the way around. In fact, there are a few inspirational ways that anxiety has helped me to elevate my life:

- Got me actively involved in personal development
- Taught me how to think in the present and act now
- Got me reading more books and discover how it heals the mind
- Started me on tracking my success and not just on failure
- Taught me how to make a positive game out of my life
- Assisted me to take control over my life
- Reconnected me to the habit of learning new things every day
- Showed me the power of meditation and visualization
- Allowed me to see that I am not the only one in my life that suffers from degrees of anxiety
- Has taught me to be a more actively vulnerable person

Using Anxiety to Your Advantage

Believe it or not, anxiety can be used for good and can be a powerful force in motivating yourself to achieve your desires. Using stress to add momentum to your life is constructive, instead of allowing it to deconstruct our lives.

Redefining danger

You must learn to see anxiety differently; anxiety, before our brains get a hold of it and dwell, is just a warning sign used for our survival. At this point, you are allowing anxiety to make you feel panicked. But even when that warning sign lights up, it doesn't mean you are in danger. You must save this energy for when you really need to make quick decisions.

Create a list of less to most dangerous to help identify a good spectrum of threats. With that comparison, you will be able to see what "dangerous" situations are safe and which ones are frightening.

Channel your stress properly

Diamonds don't grow from trees; they are coals that turn into something more beautiful through pressure. Channeling stress positively into energy for motivation does take time and can be physically and emotionally draining. But instead of allowing negative thoughts take hold of you and send you down that same spiraling hole of anxiety, look at the situation before you differently; view it as your time to *shine*! When negativity starts to manifest in your mind, challenge those thoughts. When you challenge them, you will find that the negativity in them is totally empty in the first place.

Stop trying to do your best

There are two kinds of people: those that do their best and those that can *do better*. However, those that strive to do their best constantly are the ones that end up emotionally drained than those who do better. Why? Because when you do your best, you are settling. When you strive to *do better,* you accept that you are not doing as good as you know you can. For anxiety sufferers, what they do isn't good enough for them. They either drown in their shortcomings or have learned to take the opportunity to improve themselves.

In those with anxiety, underestimation is a common cognitive distortion. When we tell ourselves that we can do better, we know how to reject our deficiencies and go out of their way to prove themselves wrong.

Chapter 8: Battling anxiety like a true warrior

"The only thing we have to fear is fear itself."

- *President Theodore Roosevelt*

Marines, SEALs, and Special Forces have no choice but to face life-threatening danger head-on regularly. The fact is, if they do get caught up in fear, they are more likely to lose their lives. While many of us will thankfully never have to face these experiences, why aren't we using the fear-crushing tactics that they use in our own personal lives?

Spend time preparing

If you are worried about a work presentation, stressing over a job interview, or freaking out about the upcoming rap battle that might help you move out of your mom's house, then stop, prepare, and practice instead of sitting around. The key is to lose yourself in the moment, which you to by devoting a ton of energy into preparing for what you are worried about. Spend 75% preparing and 25% for the actual event.

SEALs are able to erase fear by practicing upcoming mission until they feel naturally confident. When the unknown becomes more known to them, they don't have to lie to themselves about the risks, but instead put themselves in a better position to handle the unknown, which develops confidence.

Learn to *manage* fear

One of the best ways to deal with fear is to laugh about it. What? You read that right! Laughter lets you know that things are going to be okay and work out. Don't worry; there is evidence to back this theory up. A study by Stanford University showed that those that were trained to make jokes to respond to negative images. This is a much healthier way to deal with fear. The world is an inevitably twisted place, so seeing the funnier side of things makes it easier to deal with.

Breathe

When your heart is beating from your chest, your joints turn into Jell-O, and sweat is pouring off your face, then the best thing you can do to calm the physical manifestations of fear derived from anxiety is to breathe.

That simple? YES. By just inhaling for four seconds and exhaling for four seconds, SEALs can calm their nervous systems and maintain control of their natural biological responses to fear.

You are essentially bending your body's software to better control the hardware. In other words, you are giving yourself a pretty bomb superpower! Breathing helps the body go from the fight-or-flight response of the sympathetic nervous system to the relaxed response of the parasympathetic nervous system.

Tactical breathing used by Navy SEALS for performance just prior to a tense situation or during a workout:

Breathe through the nose. It's very important to breathe through your nose since breathing through the nose stimulates nerve cells that exist behind sternum near the spine that triggers the parasympathetic nervous system. Anxiety is a sympathetic response and parasympathetic counteracts that. This calms your body, which then calms your mind.

1. Relaxed sitting position and right handle on the belly.
2. Activate the breath by pushing belly out and then inhale deeply for a count of four. Inhale to the belly. This pulls breath deep into the lungs. Exhale through the nose for a count of four, pulling the belly button toward the spine. Repeat this three times.
3. Now breathe in through belly and diaphragm for a count of four, again inhaling into your belly and this time lifting your chest. Again, exhale

for a count of four so that your rib cage falls and your belly button pulls toward your spine. Repeat three times.

4. Next, use the same technique, this time inhaling for a count of four through the belly, diaphragm and your chest, with a slight raise of shoulders for inhaling. Exhale for a count of four three the chest, diaphragm, and then the belly. Repeat three times, eventually working your breaths up to eight counts.

Next, box breathing is a technique used by the U.S. Navy SEALS to maintain focus and to calm nervous system after a tense situation, such as combat, an intense workout or anytime the desire is to center and focus.

Trains for diaphragmic breathing or deep breathing. Relaxes the whole system and provides oxygen to the brain to focus better. Improves energy. It can also be used by you to regain your sense of balance, concentration, and relaxation and can be practiced at any time. Use the same technique as tactical breathing but you use a five-count hold between breaths.

1. Get in a relaxed sitting position
2. Inhale deeply through the nose for five seconds
3. Hold the air in your lungs for five seconds
4. Exhale for five seconds, releasing all the air from your lungs
5. Hold your lungs empty for five seconds
6. Repeat for five minutes, or as long as you feel necessary

Don't keep things bottled up

Fear is just like terrible liquor; it sucks when you drink it and has negative effects that last a long time, which is why it is important to deal with it before and after the fact.

Talking about scary experiences helps soldiers locate the meaning behind it all. This communication allows them to process what they have been through positively and helps them to create closer relationships with their mates. Scared? Admit it to a friend. Hearing it out loud can help you pull it out, confront it, and deal with it.

Overpower that inner nagging voice

We are all aware of the inner chatter that occurs in our mind on a daily basis. In fact, our inner voice can be really negative the majority of the time. Wouldn't it be cool to have an inner monologue that reminds us how confident and awesome we are? Wouldn't it be great to have an inner motivational speaker to get us through tough times?

Well, you can. In times of stress, our brains are wired to create self-talk that can increase our feelings of fear. As a soldier, they are expected to fight against their inner self-talk and focus on positive portions of experiences. With practice, they are easily able to ignore or even erase the negativity their brains are throwing at them. So, you can do the same in your own life.

Fear and anxiety thrive when we imagine the worst. We developed imagination to be able to project into the future so we can plan ahead. However, a side effect of being able to imagine possible positive futures is being able to imagine things going wrong. A bit of this is useful; after all, there really might be muggers or loan sharks. But uncontrolled imagination is a testing ground for anxiety and fear that can spoil otherwise happy lives.

Some people misuse their imagination chronically and so suffer much more anxiety than those who either future-project their imaginations constructively or who don't tend to think about the future much at all. Anxious, chronic worriers tend to misuse their imaginations to the extent that upcoming events feel like catastrophes waiting to happen. No wonder whole lives can be blighted by fear and anxiety.

Think of the worst-case scenario

No matter what you are afraid of, you always have the opportunity to avoid it for the rest of your life. However, soldiers don't get that choice. They face similar situations time and time again that scare them. To ensure fear doesn't overrule them, they simulate stressful scenarios and try to experience the emotions with them as well.

Instead of thinking happy thoughts and ignoring what you are afraid of, start looking at the worst things that can possibly happen. When you are able to picture the worst fear and stay within an emotional experience instead of pushing yourself out of it, your mind tends to get over the fear naturally.

Reframe your mindset

Reframe you definition of symptoms. Reframe the symptoms of anxiety - give them a different meaning. Those sweaty palms, racing heart, and lightheadedness can mean a panic attack or they can mean the most exciting and fun adventure of your life! Your body doesn't know the difference and it is just doing what it does by nature, but you can choose how you define that sudden rush. Don't believe me?

How do you think those adrenaline junkies dives off cliffs, jump motorcycles or swim with sharks? Their definition of what we call fear is definitely different. They still experience the same potent chemicals coursing through their body, but the sensations have a different meaning to them. What you experience as fear, dread and near death can be defined as thrilling, exciting, and aliveness to someone else.

The beautiful thing about consistently and purposely redefining these symptoms is you can actually rewire your brain. This leads us to neuroplasticity.

Neuroplasticity

Neuroplasticity occurs with changes in behavior, thinking, and emotions. With conscious practice, we can alter our neural pathways to move naturally towards our desired emotions, such as being thankful, calm, and happy and away from anger, stress, and panic.

As you choose to respond with positive emotion, you can strengthen the neural pathways to the desired emotions. As you make more neural connections over time to your desired emotion, the pathways to the negative reactions eventually become weaker and scrambled. This even works while using mental rehearsals of the situation and practicing your desired response.

Remember, this can also work in reverse. If you have a habitual response to circumstances, such as being angry in a traffic jam and you repeat these responses over and over in a high state of emotion, you will strengthen the neural pathways towards the emotion of anger in that situation. The masters over the centuries who taught positive thinking and faith may have actually been on to something and now we can prove it scientifically.

Get moving

Exercise is usually associated with weight loss, improved physical health, and a stronger immune system. But the benefits of exercise can expand much more. Exercise is just as important for your mental fitness as it is your physical health. Aerobic activity promotes the release of endorphins that are released in the brain and act as painkillers, which also help to increase a sense of well-being. Endorphins also improve energy levels, provide a better night's sleep, elevate your mood and provide anti-anxiety effects. Exercise also takes your mind off of your worries and breaks the cycle of negative thoughts that contribute to anxiety.

It is recommended to perform 30 minutes or more of exercise five days a week to have a significant impact on anxiety symptoms. You don't need a formal exercise program at the gym to experience these benefits. Light physical activity has been shown to have the same effects, including gardening, housework, washing the car and walking around the block. These can be done in small intervals throughout the day.

It's more important to do some sort of physical activity on a consistent basis than to aim for something that is not sustainable. Be realistic and if you need to start with smaller goals, do so. This is all about taking care of yourself in a way that works for you.

The single, most important natural tool you can use to beat anxiety is regular exercise. It sounds cliché, but the truth is that exercise affects the mind and body in ways that science is still discovering.

There is a reason that anxiety prevalence has grown with our increasingly inactive lifestyles. Jogging every day can make a world of difference in how you deal with stress, how your anxiety symptoms manifest, and how you regulate your mood.

The best methods of exercise to combat anxiety are:

- **Running** releases feel-good hormones that have exponential mental health benefits. It can help you fall asleep faster, improve memory, lower stress levels, and protects against developing depression.

- **Hiking** in a wooded or hilly location has natural calming effects on the brain. Being around plants and Earthly sights helps to reduce anxiety thanks to the chemicals plants emit. Plus, being out in nature is great for your health and memory function.

- **Yoga,** a lot like meditation, has been found to significantly reduce anxiety and other neurotic symptoms that can lead to irritability and depression. It not only strengthens your core but helps you to focus on breathing, which is the key to relaxing the mind and combating anxiety.

Chapter 9: Rediscovering yourself after hurricane anxiety

Those that live with and through the darkness of anxiety can find themselves waking up each day unhappy. Life is short and there comes a time where re-evaluating your life in order to revamp parts of it to ensure your happiness and fulfillment.

We all get lost in life from time to time. We forget old passions we had, give up interest in pursuit of something else, etc. But it is never too late to rediscover what makes you great and what makes you feel truly alive.

When were you the *happiest*?

Take a moment to remember when you were the most content with your life. In high school? College? Before marriage, family, and kids? When you began your family? Started your business? Pursued a new hobby?

No one peaks at the same time or levels in their lives. The key to regaining contentment is not to think of those fond times as "the past", but to figure out how to find that feeling of happiness again where you currently are in your life. How can you re-incorporate those things that brought you joy in the life you are living now?

What makes you *unhappy*?

What makes your blood pressure shoot through the roof? Figuring out the things that push your last buttons is just as important as knowing what helps you keep a positive outlook. When you are able to clearly point out the toxic influences, you will be better able to erase them and develop better, healthier ways of living. We tend to hold onto things from the past that has negative impacts on our current lives. What grudges are you holding onto? These are toxic and are keeping you from being your best self! No matter what it is, from a toxic ex-partner to a job that drains you, cutting these negative influences will allow you ample space to grow in a positive direction.

Write!

When negative thoughts are constantly bouncing around the brain, it can be very easy to become overwhelmed. We tend to forget how much our daily thoughts impact our lives. They take hold of our power, telling us who we are and what are and aren't capable of. We are the only ones that have the power to take action to erase pesky thoughts from inhibiting our success in life.

I have found that organizing thoughts by writing them down makes them more abstract. When you can visualize them on paper, it makes them concrete.

Write out a list of pros and cons, random thoughts that pop up, poetry, grocery lists, anything that comes to mind. All writing can be therapeutic and helps us to rediscover how our voice sounds, which radiates who. I challenge to find yourself again with the power of good old pen and paper.

Learning to Love Yourself Again

To rediscover yourself, you need to learn how to love yourself again for who you are, and all parts of yourself, including your flaws and everything you have endured. There are millions of places that offer up 'good advice' to practice self-love, but they never explain exactly how to do so.

Loving yourself is a vital piece of the puzzle when it comes to positive personal growth. It allows us to fulfill our dreams and create happy and healthy relationships with others too.

Care about yourself as much as you care about others

This sounds almost too simple, but many of us are not selfish enough when it comes to fulfilling our wants and needs. It is hard to remember that you are ***not*** selfish when it comes to caring about yourself and your wellbeing.

Showing yourself compassion shows those in your life that you are able to take care of yourself. No one can pour from an empty pot, which means you need to take care of yourself in order to take care of others in your life. Treat yourself the way you treat your best friend, with caring, concern, and gentleness, no matter what is happening in your life.

Maintain boundaries

Jot down a list of things you need emotionally, both what is important to you and what upsets you. The list can be made up of anything, from wanting sympathy to being celebrated, to being cared for, etc. Whatever is important to you, no matter how silly it sounds, ***Write. It. Down.***

We can often find ourselves smack dab in the middle of the confusing conflict and wonder how we got there in the first place. We ask ourselves how we attracted this situation and the people in it with us. While you still need to take responsibility for your actions, it is also crucial to not fall into a pit of self-blame that can cause stress, but rather really look into what is occurring. Many people lack inner confidence and have no idea what they are worth. This lack can leave us living in a sum-zero equation; we are loved completely or become completely unlovable.

I have found from my psychological studies and personal experiences that there are two very simple questions to help anyone restore healthy boundaries in their life to live a dignified life:

What does this situation negatively represent about yourself? How are you tolerating situations and the behaviors of those around you reinforces your low-worth within you? Those in our lives are a mirror of our own biases, hopes, and fears. *"All anger stems from anger at the self."*

What is your worst fear about saying "no"? Have you ever been left with the thought of you are a bad person because someone's behavior has left you feeling guilty? Well, stop! Challenge that thought by thinking about other situations you have been through. When that happens, the thought that you are a "bad person" falls apart. What matters, in the end, is simple math: people will either *add* or *subtract* to your life.

So, what have you written? The things you write are what you should consider your personal boundaries. When someone ignores something on that list, you should consider it as them crossing boundaries that you have respectively set for yourself. Do not ignore how you feel if this happens, for they are there to tell you what is right from wrong.

Inform others about the boundaries you have set for yourself and be forthcoming with what you will and will not tolerate. When you are assertive with your boundaries, this plays an important part in building a positive self-esteem and allows you many opportunities to reinforce your beliefs, what you cherish, and what you deserve from life.

Do YOU?

Take the time for yourself to establish the things that make you feel good about yourself and about your life as a whole, no matter what it is. Just learn to be aware of how you feel when you go about acting on certain things. For example:

- Are you exhausted by the work you do, but feel thrilled when gardening?
- Are you joyful when reading out loud to your children?
- Do you feel a sense of fulfillment when you write poetry or volunteer in your community?

Once you figure out what makes you feel good about yourself, make those things a priority by implementing them into your every day or weekly schedule. No matter what makes sure you go out and do them! This may mean you have to give up other things to make time for them, but it also means that you may need to re-evaluate your schedule and life more so that you are doing what you honestly enjoy.

To ensure that you are doing these things, there are more than likely going to have to be actions you take to get to those happiness goals, such as saving money to buy supplies to paint, waking up an hour earlier, exercising more, etc.

It is important to realize that you need to do what you need to in order to fulfill your happiness goals. You cannot allow yourself to blame others if you do not fulfill these things. It is time to be a little selfish and fill up your own teapot so that you can fill up the cups of others in your life! This will help you to not only feel better and do better by other people, but it will help you to clear the fog on inconsistent negativity from your life and enable you to truly love yourself and your life once more.

Conclusion:

The Path to Wellness serves as a guidebook to integrating some of the most overlooked, yet most crucial, elements of human well-being into your daily life. By providing explanations of mindfulness, chakras, and energy healing, along with an 8-week journal prompt curriculum and 50 mini-meditations, this book provides you with all the tools you need to unlock your fullest potential and deepest joy in life. The book sheds a light on the factors of well-being which are largely ignored by society, and the implications these factors have on people's mental, physical, and spiritual well-being. Complete with the ins and outs of each topic in comprehensive format, the book serves as an easy-to-follow introduction to the topics of mindfulness, chakras, and energy healing in the pursuit of holistic health. The daily guided meditations and journal prompts provided will help to bring you in touch with yourself and help you develop a larger understanding of the topics at hand. The 5- mini-meditations provided throughout the book may be integrated as needed throughout the day to regulate your energies and bring yourself into the present moment. It is our hope that this book provided you with information beyond the general scope of mental and physical wellness by drawing a map to your inner self and the deeper roots of struggle within human life. Additionally, we hope after reading this book you feel armed with both the insight and the tools to activate mindfulness, chakra knowledge, and energy healing in order to start living your best and most balanced life.

CPSIA information can be obtained
at www.ICGtesting.com
Printed in the USA
BVHW061110291221
625126BV00012B/199

9 781913 710361